THE HORMONE BALANCE COOKBOOK

To all the women out there who struggle to find well-being and balance in life. And to all of you who are suffering in silence—please seek help and don't give up. There is always a way!

MIA LUNDIN

First published by Bonnier Fakta, Stockholm, Sweden

10 9 8 7 6 5 4 3 2
Library of Congress Cataloging-in-Publication Data is available on file.

PHOTOGRAPHY BY **ULRIKA POUSSETTE**
GRAPHIC DESIGN BY **KAI RISTILA**
ILLUSTRATIONS BY **KERSTIN NORD**

PRINT ISBN: 978-1-5107-2349-8
EBOOK ISBN: 978-1-5107-2352-8

Printed in the United States of America

THE HORMONE BALANCE COOKBOOK

60 ANTI-INFLAMMATORY RECIPES TO REGULATE HORMONAL BALANCE, LOSE WEIGHT, AND IMPROVE BRAIN FUNCTION

—

TEXT: MIA LUNDIN

RECIPES: ULRIKA DAVIDSSON
PHOTOS: ULRIKA POUSETTE
TRANSLATION BY GUN PENHOAT

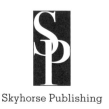

Skyhorse Publishing

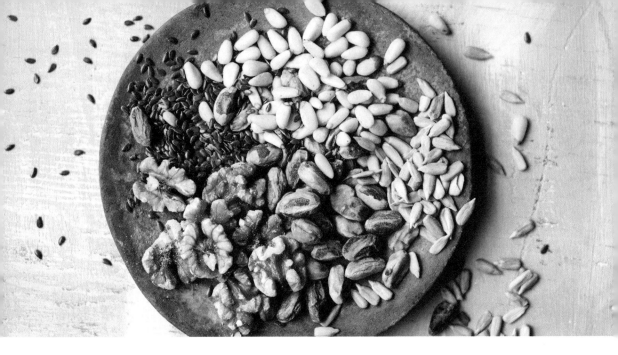

CONTENTS

FOREWORD : THE RIGHT DIET PROVIDES THE NUTRITION YOUR HORMONES NEED
Mia Lundin 4

ABOUT HORMONES 8
Are you losing your mind? 8
Your wonderfully interconnected body 9
Different types of hormones 10
The female sex hormones 11
Neurotransmitters 12
Serotonin and estrogen—a dynamic duo 13
Nutrients for serotonin production 13
Not enough food, or the wrong food 14
Your hormonal journey—from normal levels
    to menopause 15
The four hormonal phases 15
Phase 1: Normal hormonal balance 15
Phase 2: PMS—cyclically "crazy" 16
Phase 3: Perimenopause—no two days
    are alike 16
Phase 4: Menopause and postmenopause—
    where did life's joys go? 17
Where are you on your journey? 18
Do you suffer from hormonal imbalance? 18
Good nutrition goes a long way 19
Make sure to eat foods that . . . 19

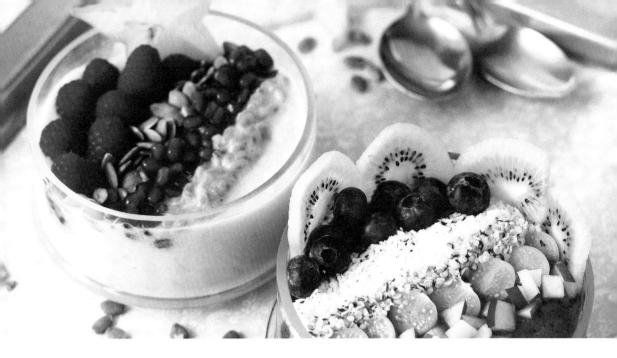

HORMONAL BALANCE 20

1. Food—the building blocks for hormones
   and a brain in balance 20
   Fat 21
   Protein 22
   Carbohydrates 23
   Minerals 25
   Vitamins 27
2. Avoid inflammation 30
   Stress and inflammation 31
   Increase your intake of
   anti-inflammatory food 31
3. Balance your blood glucose 32
   Opt for slow-release carbohydrates! 33
4. Keep your gut happy 34
   Leaky gut syndrome 34
   Dysbiosis 35
   Common Symptoms of Dysbiosis 36
   Dysbiosis and estrogen dominance 36
   Modify your eating habits 36
5. Trim your digestion 38
   A sign of good digestion 38
6. Lower your stress 39
   What makes you happy? 39
   Meditation, yoga, and breathing 40

Bioidentical Hormones 41
   Bioidentical estrogen 42
   Bioidentical progesterone 42
   Hormone replacement therapy 42
Summary, diet lists, and tables 44
   Practical diet tips—a summary 44
   Include these foods in your diet 44
   Avoid these foods 45
   Examples of ingredients for hormonal
   balance 47
   Nutritional deficiencies and their
   symptoms 48

**RECIPES: FOOD THAT IS GOOD FOR YOU
AND YOUR HORMONES 50**
Ulrika Davidsson 51
Breakfasts 52
Salads and warm soups 76
Main dishes 114
Desserts 142
A two-week diet plan 157

GLOSSARY 160
INDEX 162
SOURCES 164
CONVERSION CHARTS 166

FOREWORD: THE RIGHT DIET PROVIDES THE NUTRITION YOUR HORMONES NEED

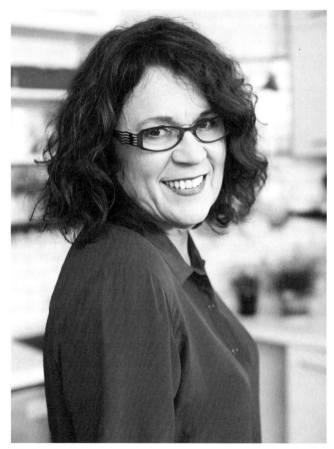

Mia Lundin

Your body is a well-functioning, intelligent machine, but it needs the right kind of fuel to work properly. By providing it with the nutrients it needs, you can prevent hormonal imbalances experienced by eight in ten perimenopausal or menopausal women. Proper nutrition goes a long way in getting rid of the problems entirely, or at least it alleviates many of the negative symptoms.

In this book, I will focus on the food and nutrients that will maintain your body's natural hormonal balance for as long as possible, and that will also keep your brain happy and sharp. You will also learn about the food that can cause hormonal imbalances.

If you've read my first book, *Female Brain Gone Insane: An Emergency Guide for Women Who Feel Like They Are Falling Apart*, or if you follow me on Facebook or read my blog, you'll know that I endorse the use of bioidentical hormones in perimenopause and menopause and for the treatment of PMS (premenstrual syndrome). Whether you're already planning on using hormone replacement therapy, or you're not yet on the journey from ordinary hormone levels to menopause and beyond, I recommend that you first build a solid foundation with balanced nutrition through food. If hormone therapy is not an option for you (perhaps due to breast cancer or past blood clots), it's even more important to focus on providing your body with the right nutrients to lessen the symptoms caused by hormonal imbalance.

I am a certified registered nurse, and a certified nurse practitioner specializing in gynecology and obstetrics. I have treated thousands of women suffering from PMS, postpartum depression, perimenopause, and menopause since 1989, focusing mainly on how hormonal imbalances affect brain chemistry.

I ran my own private clinic, the Center for Hormonal and Nutritional Balance, in California for seventeen years, where my employees and I used functional medicine (see p. 9) as the foundation for treating patients with chronic fatigue syndrome, depression, or hormonal imbalances.

> *Your body is a well-functioning, intelligent machine, but it needs the right kind of fuel to work properly.*

Our team consisted of a nutritionist, a psychologist, an NLP (neuro-linguistic programming) therapist, and me. Together, we looked at all aspects of health, physiological and psychological, and offered treatment, support, and education to enable our patients to find their way back to a place of balance, well-being, and vitality.

At my clinic, we also worked extensively on our patients' diets. It wasn't only about which foods they ate, but also about what their bodies would absorb. Did their gastrointestinal tract produce enough enzymes, gastric acid, and bile to break down all the food particles into smaller nutritional molecules that pass through the intestinal wall and into the blood? Or did most of the nutrients go straight through the body to end up in the toilet?

I met Ulrika Davidsson when I was invited to give a seminar on hormones and women's health at her restaurant on the Swedish island of Gotland. It didn't take long for us to realize that we had a lot in common, and that we might be able to help a lot of women if we published a book about food for hormonal balance. Ulrika has worked on diet, nutrition, and health for many years and has a great knowledge base in those fields. Combining her expertise with my years of experience, I knew we could write a great, accessible book for any woman who wished to take charge of her physical and emotional life.

Sooner or later, most women will experience some hormonal imbalance. Perhaps you're currently in good health, have lots of energy, and feel hormonally balanced, but still wish to support your body, mental health, and hormone production for as long as possible. Or perhaps you feel depressed, hormonally imbalanced, and exhausted due to overwhelming demands at home or at work. Either way, this book is for you.

The book is divided into two parts: a section about the facts and science, written by me, and a recipe section created by Ulrika. At the beginning of the facts section, I'll go over the different types of hormones, your sensitive hormonal system, what can cause imbalances, and various symptoms you might experience. Next, I'll explain what you should eat to provide your body with the essential nutrients that promote the production of important hormones. I'll also touch on other key topics, one of which is very close to my heart: bioidentical hormones.

" "

*Sooner or later,
most women will
experience hormonal
imbalance.*

" "

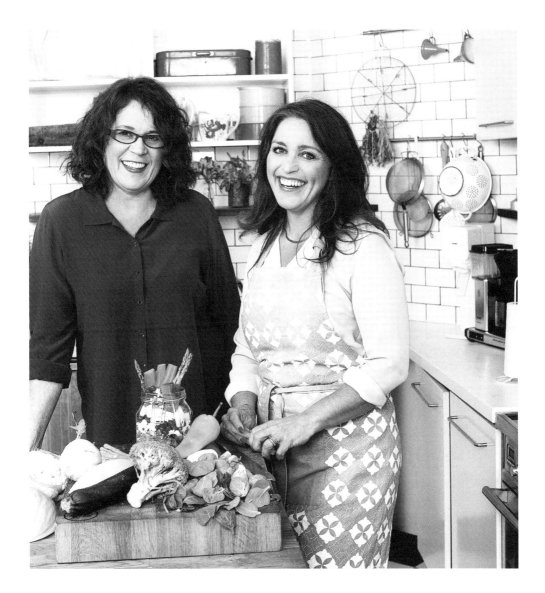

The book's first section concludes with a summary, lists of foods to include in your diet and foods to avoid, and a table of various nutritional deficiencies and their symptoms. Then you'll find Ulrika's large collection of recipes for long-lasting health and hormonal balance, plus her practical two-week meal plan to shift your production of hormones and neurotransmitters into high gear.

Finally, I want to tell you how excited I am to have the opportunity to teach you about the nutrients your body needs to bring you back to hormonal balance, vitality, and joy.

Mia Lundin (on the left) has written the book's section on facts and Ulrika Davidsson (on the right) has created the recipe section.

ABOUT HORMONES

Hormones are the body's chemical messengers. Here, we're going to look a little closer at how they interact with the brain's neurotransmitters. At the end of this section, you will learn about the four hormonal phases of a woman's life.

ARE YOU LOSING YOUR MIND?

Do you feel like you're losing your mind or going crazy? Are you on an emotional roller coaster, where one minute you're lashing out at people and the next you're crying, in desperate need of comfort and support? Perhaps you often feel low, sad, or anxious, and you can't really figure out why. You find it hard to sleep at night, and your memory plays tricks on you. Naturally, feeling this way will affect you, your family, your relationships, your career, and your ability to have fun and relax. Perhaps you believe, like many women, that your problems aren't real, and so you try to ignore them or put up with them. You might blame yourself and feel guilty, stupid, and worthless.

No, you're not losing your mind—and you don't need to feel guilty, stupid, or worthless! These problems are extremely common in women between ages thirty-five and fifty-five, because that's when hormone levels fluctuate a lot, leading to PMS (premenstrual syndrome) or symptoms of perimenopause or menopause. You're certainly not alone: over 80 percent of women in this age group suffer from these hormonal fluctuations on emotional, as well as physical, levels.

Suffering from emotional symptoms isn't a sign of personal weakness or a lack of character, any more than suffering from physical symptoms is. A woman will seek treatment if she suffers from diabetes or thyroid problems and will take insulin or thyroid medication without a second thought; however, when suffering from depression or anxiety, many women feel ashamed. It's time to stop feeling guilty and worthless. Learn about the true reason you're not feeling well: your hormones are simply out of balance. There are solutions!

YOUR WONDERFULLY INTERCONNECTED BODY

Sadly, there are still obstacles within the health and medical care community when it comes to understanding the connection between women's hormones and their mental health; many women aren't taken seriously, and they don't receive the help they should be getting.

The health care system divides the body into different specialties: neurology, cardiology, gastroenterology, gynecology, and psychiatry. Specialists focus on their respective areas of expertise and the corresponding body parts. Consequently, women seeking help for symptoms related to nutritional deficiencies and hormonal imbalance often fall in between these fields. A cardiologist will treat an irregular heartbeat and elevated blood pressure; the neurologist will check out the headache; the gastroenterologist will see to the acid reflux, IBS (irritable bowel syndrome), and gastritis; the psychiatrist will prescribe antidepressants; and the gynecologist will provide contraceptive pills and synthetic hormones.

But who's exploring potential nutritional deficiencies and hormonal imbalances? Who's looking at the full picture? Today, very few physicians have the qualifications to do this, and that's why a prescription is often the only thing given to block those symptoms. We've forgotten how to restore the body's functions in a natural way, and to create a balance between the hormones and the brain's neurotransmitters (i.e., neurochemistry).

If we really want to help patients stay healthy, a new strategy has to be introduced to our health care system. That's where functional medicine and nutritional medicine enter the scene. The body should be examined and treated in its entirety, not like a container of separate parts. Instead of seeing a patient as merely a collection of different organs, we need to start looking at how the body works together as one whole unit!

Functional and nutritional medicine are based on the principle that we should try to restore the original function of the organ or the biochemical processes before an imbalance deteriorates into illness. For example, your body needs nutrients, such as amino acids and vitamins, to manufacture signal substances. If you don't supply your body with what it needs, there will be an imbalance between the signal substances, making you feel anxious or depressed. Instead of taking medication, which only suppresses the symptoms, practitioners of functional medicine recommend that you give your body the nutrients it needs. This way, you're treating the underlying source of the problem using a natural approach, not just masking the symptom.

"The body should be examined and treated in its entirety, not like a container of separate parts."

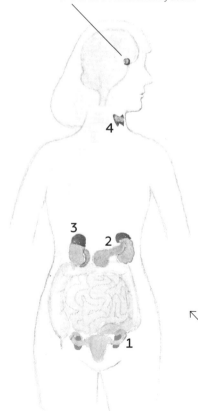

You must have hormonal equilibrium at all stages of life to feel well and to prevent illness.

The pituitary gland regulates the entire hormonal system

If you want to be healthy and prevent illnesses, such as osteoporosis, cardiovascular disease, and depression, you must have hormonal equilibrium at all stages of life. This becomes especially important around ages thirty-five to fifty, when hormones fluctuate and you're more easily impacted by stress and poor diet. Having too many or too few hormones may contribute to a host of different problems that will make you feel out of sorts.

The good news is that there's a lot you can do yourself. You lay the foundation for your own well-being and keep yourself healthy by eating the right types of food according to your body's needs. When you provide your body with the nutrients it's been clamoring for, it will stop crying out for help, which in turn will make you feel calm and collected. The more nutritionally balanced your body is, the fewer hormones you'll need to replace when the time comes, and the less you'll suffer from premenstrual symptoms as you enter perimenopause or menopause.

DIFFERENT TYPES OF HORMONES

Hormones are your body's natural signal molecules that regulate different functions on a cellular level, and by extension, your well-being. Those signals have to work well for you to feel good.

Several different glands in the body produce hormones, such as the ovaries, the thyroid, the adrenal glands, and the pancreas. Hormones travel through the bloodstream until they reach specific cells—the target cells they influence.

Our ovaries produce estrogen, progesterone, and testosterone, which regulate ovulation, fertility, and sex drive; the thyroid hormones thyroxine (T4) and triiodothyronine (T3) regulate metabolism; the adrenal hormones cortisol and adrenaline regulate stress and immune defense; and the pancreas's insulin stores energy. In this book, we'll concentrate primarily on the female sex hormones.

GLANDS THAT PRODUCE HORMONES

1. ovaries
2. pancreas
3. adrenal glands
4. thyroid

THE FEMALE SEX HORMONES

Estrogen: During your fertile years, your ovaries produce three different types of estrogen: estradiol, estrone, and estriol. Much scientific research has shown that estradiol is important for brain function. Estradiol increases blood flow to the brain and keeps it sharp. It even works as a type of natural antidepressant, and stabilizes your mood by keeping the serotonin and dopamine (see p. 12–13) transmitters at good levels. Estradiol also has an anti-inflammatory effect that protects blood vessels against plaque formation.

Estrone, produced in the ovaries and the fat cells, is the type of estrogen we have the most of after menopause. However, it doesn't have any obvious effect on menopausal symptoms.

Estriol is secreted in large quantities from the placenta during pregnancy. However, it's a relatively weak estrogen that doesn't affect emotional symptoms or cause many hot flashes or sleep disturbances. It can be used as a topical treatment in the vagina, as a cream or suppositories to decrease dryness, stinging, and irritation, and it can be purchased without a prescription at the drugstore.

Progesterone, produced in the corpus luteum (Latin for "yellow body"), is the first hormone that decreases as you age. By the middle to end of your thirties, it starts to drop along with decreasing ovulation, and often with increasing stress levels.

Very low levels of progesterone cause PMS (premenstrual syndrome, see p. 16) and menopausal problems. Progesterone doesn't seem to be quite as important for brain function as estrogen, but it does have a calming effect on mood since it increases the level of the soothing neurotransmitter GABA (Gabapentin) in the brain. Progesterone also increases the amount of serotonin receptors in the brain

ESTROGEN
- keeps the brain sharp
- stabilizes mood
- has an anti-inflammatory effect

PROGESTERONE
- calms the nervous system
- calms mood

HORMONE LEVELS DURING THE MENSTRUAL CYCLE

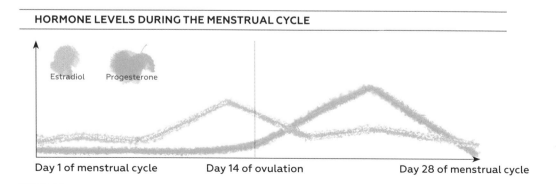

Estradiol   Progesterone

Day 1 of menstrual cycle   Day 14 of ovulation   Day 28 of menstrual cycle

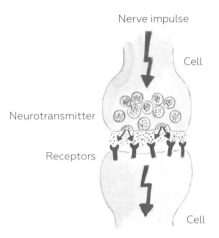

Nerve impulse

Cell

Neurotransmitter

Receptors

Cell

SYNAPSE

When a nerve impulse reaches the synapse, neurotransmitters are released and trigger the next cell through its receptors. The cell on the receiving end is stimulated and generates a new impulse, which then continues on to the next cell.

and the sensitivity of these receptors. With enough progesterone during the second half of the menstrual cycle, the body has better access to the calming neurotransmitters GABA and serotonin. This explains why women who suffer from PMS often feel irritated and anxious. On the other hand, while progesterone calms the nervous system, too much of it can cause fatigue, sleepiness, or even slight depression.

NEUROTRANSMITTERS

You've already heard of neurotransmitters, the brain's and body's chemical "messengers" that transfer information from one brain cell to another and make it possible for the brain cells to communicate with each other, as well as with other cells in the body.

Neurotransmitters, to a large extent, are the driving force behind your emotions, thoughts, experiences, and mood. That's why an imbalance between neurotransmitters, or a lack of certain neurotransmitters, can make you feel bad. The brain's chemicals were a mystery to us for a long time, but now we can measure their levels and influence them with natural supplements and certain foods, among other things.

To make the entire body's sophisticated and complex nervous system function and communicate the right way, impulses need to travel quickly from one cell to the next. But the nerve cells aren't attached to one another; there are small spaces between each cell called synapses. It's there, in these small spaces, that you need to have enough neurotransmitters so the impulse can travel from one cell to the next.

This process is repeated from one brain cell to the next as an impulse travels toward its ultimate destination, which makes it possible for us to move our bodies, think, feel, and communicate.

Neurotransmitters can have a soothing or a stimulating effect. Soothing neurotransmitters work like a brake pedal in your body, and their main purpose is to filter out unnecessary stimulating signals, calm the senses and body, and make you feel peaceful. They even begin the sleep cycle. Serotonin and GABA are examples of soothing neurotransmitters.

Stimulating neurotransmitters function like a gas pedal in your body, and their main purpose is to provide you with energy, motivation, and focus. Dopamine and noradrenaline are examples of stimulating neurotransmitters.

As you probably know, establishing a balance between the brake and gas pedals—between the calming and the stimulating neurotransmitters—is necessary for your well-being.

SEROTONIN AND ESTROGEN—A DYNAMIC DUO

The reason I write about neurotransmitters in a book on nutrition and hormonal balance is because neurotransmitters and hormones work closely together. In fact, I like to call the neurotransmitter serotonin and the female sex hormone estrogen a dynamic duo!

When the level of estrogen drops, so do the levels of serotonin, which can leave you feeling jumpy, anxious, and irritated. Normal and stable levels of estrogen are necessary for serotonin production and function, which in turn ensures that the ovaries produce the right level of estrogen.

It's this teamwork of hormones and neurotransmitters that is vital to your well-being and hormonal balance. What's more, you can influence the production of both hormones and neurotransmitters by following the right diet.

NUTRIENTS FOR SEROTONIN PRODUCTION

Just like a car needs the right type of fuel to work efficiently, your body needs the right nutrients to create neurotransmitters. Think about it: when you're out driving and the red gas light comes on, do you smash the light with a hammer and keep on driving? Or do you pour orange juice under the hood of your car instead of motor oil? No; you know what the problem is and you fill your car with gas to prevent the engine from stalling, or you take your car in for service.

Imagine your emotional and physical symptoms as a brightly lit red gas light on the dashboard. When you feel exhausted, anxious, gloomy, irritable, or just restless, your body and brain need the right raw materials—the right nutrients—to manufacture the right neurotransmitters and hormones. And it can be relatively simple to restore that balance once you've learned which foods to eat and which foods to avoid.

NEUROTRANSMITTERS

STIMULATING DOPAMINE/NORADRENALINE
• provides energy, motivation, and focus

CALMING SEROTONIN/GABA
• soothes mood and the body

For your body to produce neurotransmitters like serotonin, it needs raw materials from your diet, and sometimes additional nutrition in the form of dietary supplements:

• **Amino acid tryptophan** (see sources under "Good protein sources," p. 23)
• **Vitamin B6** (see sources on p. 27)
• **Folic acid (B9)** (see sources on p. 28)
• **Vitamin D** (see sources on p. 29)
• **Magnesium** (see sources on p. 25)

A WELL-NOURISHED BRAIN MAKES YOU
• alert
• happy
• focused
• organized
• less affected by stress

NOT ENOUGH FOOD, OR THE WRONG FOOD

Dieting or a nutritionally poor diet can malnourish the brain and lead to a lack of amino acids, essential vitamins, and minerals. These deficiencies slow down the production and circulation of neurotransmitters, which in turn can cause emotional problems and cravings for certain types of food—often carbohydrate-dense foods such as pastries, chocolate, and candy, as well as alcohol. A lack of the neurotransmitter dopamine diminishes feelings of satisfaction and motivation, while a lack of serotonin and GABA produces feelings of restlessness, stress, and anxiety.

Luckily, your brain reacts quickly when it gets proper nourishment. You will soon feel more alert and happy and will be better able to concentrate, organize, and function both at home and at work. You'll also be less affected by stress, and the less stressed you are, the more established the delicate balance between the brain and the ovaries will be.

Make sure to eat what your body needs to produce neurotransmitters and hormones, and avoid foods that block your hormones' work. Your intelligent body will take care of the rest.

YOUR HORMONAL JOURNEY—FROM NORMAL LEVELS TO MENOPAUSE

Unfortunately, your ovaries don't work throughout your entire lifetime. From your midthirties until your late fifties, your body undergoes many changes. Your hormone levels, especially the female sex hormones estrogen and progesterone, can fluctuate wildly, which affects the brain's neurotransmitters. Hormone production in the ovaries ceases during menopause, typically at the onset, or middle, of your fifties. But your body doesn't shut down the production overnight; the process can take ten to fifteen years. That's a long time to endure emotional and physical turmoil! That's why it's so important that you find solutions to lessen your symptoms and to make you feel healthy and happy.

Throughout your life, you'll go through four significant hormonal phases, each with its own set of possible emotional and physical indicators. Some women simply glide through these changes without any real problems, while others deal with all kinds of complications. The more nutritionally balanced you are, the fewer problems you're likely to encounter. So, don't give up even if it seems hard, and keep reading for more tips that will help you along the way.

THE FOUR HORMONAL PHASES

PHASE 1: NORMAL HORMONAL BALANCE

Naturally, we all feel slightly different every day, throughout most of our lives. When you are in this phase, which starts as you begin to menstruate, you should feel about the same over the whole month. Symptoms like nervousness, irritability, depression, and headaches don't increase drastically right before your period, which means that you *don't* suffer from PMS or hormonal imbalance. However, moodiness, anxiety, and feelings of sadness can be caused by stress and an imbalance of neurotransmitters. This can happen at all ages—and teenage girls are no exception.

The reason your hormones are in such a fine-tuned balance month after month during your years of fertility is to prepare your body

> *The reason your hormones are in such a fine-tuned balance month after month during your years of fertility is to prepare the body for pregnancy.*

for pregnancy. However, if your body is under duress—because of extreme physical demands or a poor diet, for example—your nervous system will interpret this as hazardous, which puts a stop to hormone production and ovulation. You are not meant to become pregnant when you're in acute danger.

PHASE 2: PMS—CYCLICALLY "CRAZY"

The PMS phase—premenstrual syndrome—usually starts when you're in your thirties, but it can also begin earlier in life under stressful conditions. Here, the level of the calming hormone progesterone, which is produced after ovulation, starts to drop, giving rise to heightened nervousness, anger, irritability, and depression before the start of your period. These symptoms typically last from a few days to two full weeks. This can cause a great deal of discomfort, but the symptoms disappear as soon as menstruation begins. The period itself usually remains unchanged.

PHASE 3: PERIMENOPAUSE—NO TWO DAYS ARE ALIKE

This phase often starts in your forties and can last between one and ten years; it ends when you stop menstruating. Feelings of anxiety, anger, and depression, as well as hot flashes and night sweats, might appear a few days or up to two weeks *before* menstruation. These symptoms are replaced by new ones once menstruation starts—namely fatigue, sleep disturbances, weepiness, and apathy. I've heard

THE FOUR HORMONAL PHASES

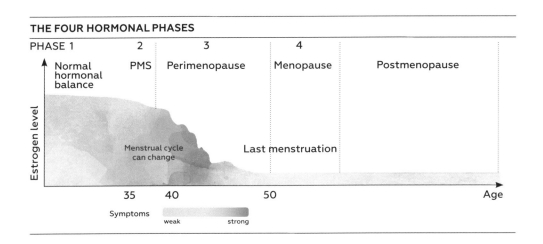

some women say that they only feel normal during one week out of the entire month during this phase. Periods can become more frequent and heavier, and they often contain clots of blood, which can lead to iron deficiency.

Symptoms in this phase are often caused by a condition called estrogen dominance—an imbalance between the amounts of estrogen and progesterone. In fact, estrogen levels can be low, normal, or high in estrogen dominance; what actually causes those symptoms is when progesterone levels are too low compared to estrogen levels, i.e., too low to balance out the effects from the estrogen. In other words, a woman with low estrogen levels can also have symptoms of estrogen dominance.

The imbalance between estrogen and progesterone in phase 3 often leads to weight gain, since estrogen stimulates breast cells to make them bigger and heavier.

Estrogen dominance can also prevent the body from processing thyroid hormones, which results in a lower metabolism and weight gain.

This imbalance also affects the body's level of fluids because progesterone, which acts as a diuretic, is now in deficit. Another reason for weight gain can be inflammation in the body (see more about this on p. 30). When there's not enough progesterone, which has an anti-inflammatory effect, the risk of inflammation increases.

> *The imbalance between estrogen and progesterone in phase 3 often leads to weight gain.*

PHASE 4: MENOPAUSE AND POSTMENOPAUSE—WHERE DID LIFE'S JOYS GO?

Menopause, also referred to as "the change," often starts around fifty years of age and typically ends about one year after your last period. Symptoms during this phase are usually similar every day. Menstruation occurs less often, perhaps only a few times in the year, or it has stopped altogether. Common symptoms in menopause are apathy, weepiness, sleep disturbances, hot flashes, heart palpitations, loss of concentration, and brain fog. You might not recognize yourself, and activities that used to bring you joy may now feel like an uninteresting chore. The ovaries are now producing very little estrogen and no progesterone at all. After menopause, you are in the postmenopausal phase, which lasts to the end of life.

HOW TO READ TEST RESULTS

Here are approximate reference values:
- Normal hormonal balance and PMS phase: 1.5–10
- Perimenopause: 11–20
- Menopause and postmenopause: above 20

WHERE ARE YOU ON YOUR JOURNEY?

Sometimes it's difficult to know which phase you're in based only on symptoms and periods. A blood test for a follicle-stimulating hormone (FSH) is a good option that will provide more clues. Take an FSH blood test sometime between the third and fifth day of menstruation. If your period has ceased or if it's erratic because you're using an intrauterine device, you need to have your blood drawn twice, with two weeks in between. You then look at the lowest FSH result of the two tests.

Perimenopause and menopause are inevitable phases on your hormonal journey. Having helped thousands of women throughout my practice, I am totally convinced that many need to take bioidentical hormone replacement to maintain not only the best health but also a good mood (read more about bioidentical hormone replacement on p. 41). Whether you take hormone replacements or not, it's important that your body gets the nutrition it needs—the healthier a diet you eat when you enter perimenopause and menopause, the fewer symptoms you will experience as your ovaries begin to retire and your estrogen levels decrease.

COMMON SYMPTOMS OF HORMONAL AND NEUROTRANSMITTER IMBALANCE

- Irritability
- Anger
- Apathy
- Jumpiness, feeling agitated
- Depression
- Anxiety
- Mood swings
- Sleep disturbances
- Weepiness
- Decreased or increased libido
- Loss of concentration
- Decreased motivation
- Weight gain

DO YOU SUFFER FROM HORMONAL IMBALANCE?

The interaction between hormones and neurotransmitters during hormonal changes throughout your life basically lays down the foundation for how you feel. Your hormones and neurotransmitters are chemical "messengers" that distribute important instructions everywhere in your body. They make sure you can function physically and mentally as a person—for example as you move around, think, feel, and communicate with others.

Your hormones are designed to function together as a whole and work as a team in sync with nature's daily biorhythms and the changing of the seasons. If, for some reason, hormone levels decrease or stop working well, you'll probably feel the effects. These symptoms are very common in women, especially those between the ages of thirty-five and fifty-five, and should be taken seriously. That said, with the dietary advice, recipes, and tips in this book, you can learn to address and solve your problems.

GOOD NUTRITION GOES A LONG WAY

Unfortunately, there's no single diet you can follow that will magically transform the food you eat into the hormones your ovaries will produce (hormone production that, by the way, will decrease over time). Many women have asked me if they should eat yams or sweet potatoes to increase progesterone in the body, since they've heard that the bioidentical progesterone in pharmacies is extracted from these root vegetables. However, note that it's only the vegetable hormone that is extracted, which is then modified in a laboratory until it becomes identical to your endogenous progesterone. In other words, nothing of the root vegetable itself is used during this extraction process, so it won't do any good to eat sweet potatoes, even if by the truckload.

Even so, with the right diet you *can* keep your hormones in balance longer and delay or lessen the symptoms of menopause.

MAKE SURE TO EAT FOODS THAT...

- contain the building blocks for your female sex hormones
- contain the nutrients you need to create neurotransmitters, which make you happier and less stressed
- decrease inflammation in your body, since inflammation causes imbalance in hormonal levels and brain chemistry
- balance your blood glucose and insulin, since a diet high in sugar causes elevated insulin levels, which in turn blocks hormone receptors and makes it more difficult for hormones to enter the cells
- keep your gut healthy with wholesome bacteria, which break down the hormones so your body can use them and then get rid of them.

Additionally, if you practice mindfulness, yoga, or meditation; socialize and laugh with your family and friends; or take hikes in the woods, you'll lower your levels of the stress hormone cortisol, which will help you relax a bit. Most important of all, you must get enough sleep. At least 7–8 hours per night is a good goal for most of us. Too little sleep increases cortisol levels, which can lead to weight gain, mood swings, fatigue, irritability, memory loss, and loss of concentration. Having increased levels of cortisol also makes it difficult to fall asleep.

As with insulin, high levels of cortisol block estrogen receptors and prevent estrogen from entering the cells. You'll find more about this in the next section, "Hormonal Balance" (p. 20).

> *Most important of all, you must get enough sleep. At least 7–8 hours per night is a good goal for most of us.*

HORMONAL BALANCE

Hormonal balance is a prerequisite for your well-being. In this part of the book, we'll go through the six most important factors— nutrition, inflammation, blood glucose, gut flora, digestion, and stress—that you can control to maintain hormonal balance as effectively and for as long as possible.

1. FOOD—THE BUILDING BLOCKS FOR HORMONES AND A BRAIN IN BALANCE

You know it's important to eat healthily. But did you know that you can also become happier and achieve hormonal balance by following a certain type of diet, and that, on the flip side, there are types of food that can cause imbalances?

What you eat affects your hormone production, brain function, mood, and, of course, your health. If your food doesn't contain the right nutrients, your body will not be able to produce hormones the right way and maintain hormonal balance since it doesn't have the means to. It's that simple.

Your body needs five basic nutritional components in your food to get everything it requires: fat, protein, carbohydrates, minerals, and vitamins.

It can't function without these nutrients; it won't recover and can't replace worn-out cells. In addition, your brain won't function optimally, which negatively affects hormone production.

YOUR BODY, BRAIN, AND HORMONES NEED:
• protein
• fat
• carbohydrates
• vitamins
• minerals

To a large extent, our emotions, thoughts, experiences, memories, and moods are steered by the brain's "messengers," the different neurotransmitters (primarily serotonin, noradrenaline, dopamine, and GABA). If their levels are disturbed due to bad food choices and stress, hormone production will also be adversely affected, giving rise to depression, sleep problems, and loss of focus.

On the other hand, if your brain gets what it needs, you'll increase your chances of feeling healthy and happy and experience a sense of well-being, which in turn can lead you to make good decisions for yourself and your life. Naturally, it's best to get the nutrition you need directly from the food you eat. Simply put, it's proper nutrition. But sometimes we have to add some dietary supplements to the mix because the food we eat today can't always provide us with all the necessary vitamins and essential amino acids—a consequence of depleted soil and overly processed ingredients, among other things.

Daily stress, contraceptive pills and some medications, alcohol, and vegetarian or vegan diets (which can contain too little protein, if one is not diligent) can also increase the body's need for certain nutrients. Eating right requires a bit of planning, which on some days is easier said than done.

Healthy food should be a part of your daily regimen, just like exercise and adequate rest, so that hormone production can proceed just as it should. The following is a list of the most important nutrients for your body, and the foods you'll find them in.

FAT

Fat is one of the most important nutrients for hormonal balance. You need fat for your well-being. Hormones are produced by certain amino acids and cholesterol, which are found in fat. If you eat too little fat, hormone production will suffer, especially the production of the female sex hormones estrogen and progesterone.

Your brain consists of 60 percent fat, and it needs the right kind of fat to function. Over the last decade neuroscientists have discovered that essential amino acids like omega-3 fatty acids, EPA (eikosapentaenoic acid), and DHA (docosahexaenoic acid), for example, are pivotal to the structure of the brain itself. The word "essential" means your body depends on these fatty acids, but it can't generate them by itself—you need to get them from the foods you eat.

Without essential fatty acids, your brain tissue starves and the nerve cells harden and shrivel up. As a result, neurotransmitters can't relay information from cell to cell, and that affects our ability to learn, focus, and recall. (Read more about neurotransmitters on p. 12.)

Our old widespread phobia of fats is ebbing—earlier beliefs about saturated fat contributing directly to high cholesterol are being questioned more and more. But what happened when we were in the grip of our nonfat hysteria? Well, we threw out all types of fats, including the wholesome omega-3 fatty acids (EPA and DHA), replacing them with faster-acting carbohydrates, such as starch and sugar. What was the outcome? More and more people became overweight and depressed.

Exercise, rest, and nutrient-rich food makes hormone production proceed like it should!

> *Balanced levels of omega-6 and omega-3 essential fatty acids are key to survival.*

SUGGESTION IF YOUR DIET IS INCOMPLETE:
· Omega-3 fish oil, per capsule
· Concentrated fish oil, 1,000 mg, which contains:
  · eikosapentaenoic acid (EPA) 300–500 mg
  · docosahexaenoic acid (DHA) 200–250 mg
· Recommended intake: 1–3 capsules daily

Make sure you buy pure fish oil, i.e., from fish that are free of impurities such as heavy metals and pesticides.

Omega-6 and omega-3 fatty acids are both key to survival. Your body can't make omega-3s or omega-6s on its own; the only way to get them is through the food you eat. That's why low-fat diets can be dangerous: they systematically rob our bodies of the fat we need to function. This is an important issue that can't be ignored!

Omega-3 fatty acids have other benefits: they reduce inflammation and prevent weight gain by increasing insulin sensitivity, i.e., they make it easier for insulin to enter the cells and balance blood glucose levels (read more about this on p. 32).

It's easier for us to get omega-6 fatty acids, which stimulate muscle growth and hormone production. However, they can cause inflammation, and, a little strangely, they compete with omega-3 acids to a certain extent.

Long before our food supply became industrialized, the food we ate provided a natural balance of these two essential fatty acids. The issue with today's Western diet is that it contains lower levels of omega-3 fatty acids than before, while supplying us with far more omega-6 fatty acids, causing an imbalance.

If you want to reduce your risk of inflammation, cut back on your intake of foods containing high amounts of omega-6 fatty acids such as grains (flour, bread, pasta), sunflower oil, corn oil, margarine, and sesame seeds.

To get more omega-3 fatty acids, concentrate on eating flaxseeds, flaxseed oil, chia seeds, pumpkin seeds, walnuts, salmon, and other fatty fish like herring and mackerel (preferably wild-caught). If you eat meat, stick to organic meat from grass-fed animals (or game). Omega-3 eggs from hens fed a special diet will also give you an extra boost of the right fats.

PROTEIN

Proteins are made up of amino acids and can be found in all body cells. Most processes in the body depend on proteins. The brain, for example, requires a certain level of amino acids to create neurotransmitters. Too little of the amino acids tyrosine and tryptophan, for example, leads to decreased levels of the neurotransmitters serotonin, dopamine, and noradrenalin, which can bring on symptoms like nervousness, anxiety, sleeping problems, and brain fog (read more about neurotransmitters on p. 12).

About twenty amino acids are required to build up our brain's chemistry, but only eleven of these are manufactured by the body. You can only obtain the rest through the food you eat and through supplements, if you take them. I recommend my patients start the day off with a protein-rich breakfast (approx. 20 g protein) and include protein at lunch and dinner. Each person's needs will vary, however, depending on your body weight and how active you are. The general daily recommendation for adults, in line with the WHO (World Health Organization), is approximately 0.8–0.9 g per kg (about 0.36 g per lb) of body weight.

Some good sources of protein are organic meat, eggs, fish, shellfish, poultry, and game. If you don't eat red meat, go for free-range chicken, turkey, and wild-caught fish. If you're vegetarian, make sure to eat lentils, seaweed, quinoa, peanut butter, chickpeas, hemp seeds, chia seeds, and almond milk.

CARBOHYDRATES

The brain's most important fuel comes from the carbohydrates we ingest; however, it is also a fuel we can't store. The body breaks down carbohydrates into sugar in the form of glucose, which is then transported to the brain and throughout the body via blood circulation and is used immediately for energy. The brain depends on glucose for many of its functions, such as the ability to think, short- and long-term memory, and sleeping.

Many diets, especially low-carbohydrate diets, promote an intake of carbohydrates that is too low; the latest research indicates that this has a negative effect on the brain's functions.

Carbohydrates also enhance the uptake of the amino acid tryptophan, which is converted to serotonin in the brain. That's why you often feel a bit calmer and more relaxed half an hour or so after eating a meal with carbohydrates, an aftereffect that usually lasts for several hours.

However, it's important to choose the right type of carbohydrates and avoid fast-acting carbohydrates that are typically found in foods like white bread, sodas, candy, pastries, chips, and pasta. Fast-acting carbohydrates give the brain a sudden jolt of sugar, which is often followed by a blood sugar crash about thirty minutes later, lowering your glucose levels more than they were before you ate. You end up feeling

> *Slow-release carbohydrates are the brain's most important fuel.*

hungry, dizzy, irritable, and tired, and will soon start craving more fast-acting carbohydrates to stave off your discomfort. This goes on and easily turns into a vicious circle. Fast-acting carbohydrates also lead to elevated insulin levels, which in turn block your estrogen's access to cells (read more about this on p. 32).

By contrast, slow-release carbohydrates are full of fiber, vitamins, and minerals, and they provide the brain with a more even stream of glucose, which improves its function. They provide more nutrients to our body and healthy gut bacteria, and even alleviate our cravings for sweets. They also help intestinal function, which can reduce the risk of constipation and even help in weight loss.

I often recommend that my patients try to avoid gluten, especially those in America (where I live), because gluten is often genetically modified in the US. It can cause brain fog and inflammation in the gut. An inflamed gut raises the level of the neurotransmitter glutamate in the brain, which can lead to racing thoughts, nervousness, and anxiety. The connection between inflammation, anxiety, and depression was discussed as far back as the 1990s, and research continues to investigate whether it's possible that anti-inflammatory medication can cure depression. (Scientists in Lund, a university town in southern Sweden, were the first to notice inflammatory changes in the spinal fluid of suicidal patients.)

SUGGESTION IF YOUR DIET IS LACKING ADEQUATE NUTRIENTS:
Magnesium 200–600 mg daily

When taking magnesium supplements, you should consider its bioavailability, i.e., how much of the magnesium is absorbed by the body. The most bioavailable forms of magnesium are magnesium glycinate, magnesium citrate, and magnesium taurate. Magnesium citrate can cause loose stools, so if that's a problem for you, choose magnesium glycinate instead. Avoid magnesium carbonate, magnesium sulfate, and magnesium gluconate, as they're more difficult for the body to absorb.

I recommend that you take the dose at bedtime, especially if you have trouble falling asleep, since magnesium is calming for both body and soul.

In my experience, if an episode of depression is caused by inflammation, the source is usually a leaky gut. When I've recommended that my patients take probiotics and fish oil, and eat fermented and other anti-inflammatory foods, their nervousness, anxiety, and depression decrease. (Read more about leaky gut on p. 34.)

Examples of good, slow-release carbohydrates include whole grain products (if you are gluten-tolerant), fruit, legumes, lentils, brown rice, quinoa, buckwheat, oats, and vegetables.

IMPORTANT MINERALS
FOR HORMONES:
• magnesium
• zinc
• selenium
• iron

MINERALS

The body is made up of approximately twenty different elements. Apart from oxygen, carbon, hydrogen, and nitrogen, the body also needs mineral elements to function. Minerals are solid, inorganic substances that are found in nature in the soil, bedrock, and water. Magnesium, zinc, selenium, and iron are examples of minerals that are important in the production of neurotransmitters and hormones.

You'd think we would get all the minerals we need by eating the right kinds of food. Unfortunately, most of the vegetables we buy today don't contain enough minerals, due in large part to the continued depletion of farmed soils. Even the level of minerals in meat is lower than it used to be. Nevertheless, game, organic meat, and organically grown vegetables often have a higher mineral content.

Magnesium is the second most lacking mineral in the Western diet—only a deficiency in vitamin D is more common. Magnesium, also called the "anti stress mineral," has a calming effect and strengthens our ability to focus. It relaxes nerves and muscles and diminishes the effects of stress. Moreover, magnesium is required to produce several of the brain's neurotransmitters. (Patients who are depressed typically exhibit low levels of magnesium.) Quite simply, magnesium is vital for the brain's and body's neurotransmitters to function properly.

A lack of magnesium gives rise to a lot of symptoms that we associate with PMS, such as irritability, depression, confusion, memory fails, menstrual pain, and muscle aches. Good sources of magnesium are leafy greens, beans, nuts, seeds, and gluten-free whole grains, among other things.

Zinc increases our ability to concentrate. Lacking this mineral can cause hair loss, fatigue, problems focusing, depression, and mood swings. Good sources of zinc are organic meat, liver, shellfish, and whole grains.

Selenium plays a valuable role in the cells' oxygen support, the nervous system, and metabolism. It is needed in the production of thyroid hormones and the neurotransmitters dopamine and serotonin. It is also very good for strong hair and nails. Older people and vegetarians often need to take a selenium supplement.

Selenium is an antioxidant that protects body cells from disintegrating. Free radicals are constantly secreted in the body, especially when we are stressed out or live unhealthily, breaking down cells and making them age prematurely. Antioxidants, like selenium, help fight this breakdown.

Good sources of selenium are fish and shellfish, such as salmon, mackerel, oysters, and mussels, along with seaweed, free-range meat, organ meats, eggs, and nuts.

Iron is vital to a lot of the body's processes. It is needed to transport oxygen through the blood vessels, as well as in the production of certain neurotransmitters such as dopamine. Iron deficiency can negatively affect faculties like attention span, logical thinking, learning, and memory. It can also lead to fatigue, apathy, breathlessness, palpitations, trouble sleeping, irritability, vertigo, nervousness, and headaches.

Heavy, irregular menstrual periods are common in the perimenopausal phase, which can lead to an iron deficiency. That's why it's particularly important during this time to eat foods that are rich in iron. Good sources of iron include grass-fed meat, spinach, leeks, green peas, sardines, and egg yolks.

VITAMINS

Many of the body's chemical processes depend on vitamins. Since the body is unable to produce vitamins by itself (except for vitamin D), you must obtain them through the food you eat. Vitamins B and C are water soluble and don't store easily in the body, which means there is an increased risk of deficiency with these vitamins. However, fat-soluble vitamins A, D, E, and K all store well in the body, over quite a long period of time. It has been shown that there is a link between depression and a lack of certain vitamins like B1, B3, B6, Folic Acid (B9), B12, C, and D.

B vitamins are important for both your mental and emotional well-being. They can't be stored in the body, which means you must take B vitamins daily through your diet to improve brain function.

Stress leads to an increased need of B vitamins. Alcohol, contraceptive pills, refined sugar, nicotine, and caffeine impair their absorption, so it isn't hard to understand why so many of us are lacking in these vitamins. Common symptoms of vitamin B deficiency are depression, anxiety, irritability, and heightened PMS.

Vitamin B1 (thiamine) is used by the brain to convert glucose (blood sugar) to fuel. When your brain is short of thiamine, it quickly loses energy, which can result in fatigue, irritability, nervousness, and depression.

Vitamin B3 (niacin) has a positive impact on memory, and it lessens the risk of depression. A lack of vitamin B3 can bring on feelings of stress and nervousness, as well as mental and physical lethargy.

Vitamin B5 (pantothenic acid) is important for hormone production and the absorption of amino acids and the neurotransmitter acetylcholine. Together they act against certain types of depression. A vitamin B5 deficiency can lead to fatigue, chronic stress, and depression.

Vitamin B6 (pyridoxine) is needed in the production of the neurotransmitters serotonin, melatonin, and dopamine. B6 is also needed for the creation of amino acids, which produce proteins that build and repair body tissues.

> *Common symptoms of vitamin B deficiency are depression, anxiety, irritability, and heightened PMS.*

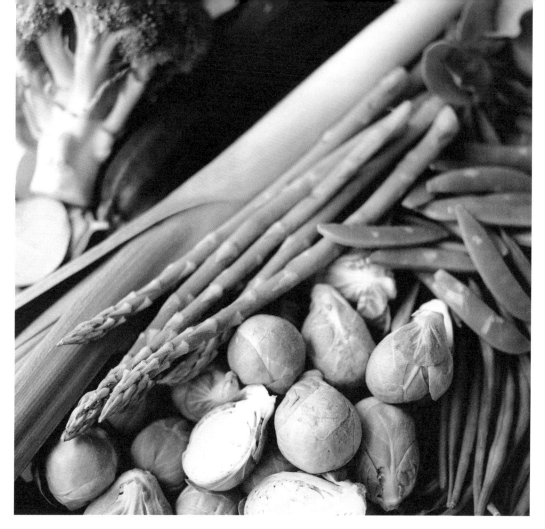

B9 (folic acid) deficiency is very common. B9 can be found in dark green vegetables, organic, grass-fed meat, fish, shellfish, milk, cheese, eggs, and liver.

Vitamin B9 (folic acid) contributes to a healthy nervous system and even moods. Bad food habits, certain illnesses, alcoholism, and some drugs (aspirin and other medications containing acetylsalicylic acid, contraceptive pills, and anti cramping preparations, for example) can cause a folic acid deficiency.

A lack of vitamin B12 can hide a folic acid deficiency, so they're often administered together. If you're low on folic acid, you're at an increased risk of depression; plus, anti depressants usually work better when taken together with folic acid. The 5-MHTF form of folic acid is best, as it is most easily absorbed by the body's cells.

Vitamin B12 (cobalamine) is required for red blood cell production and the proper functioning of the nervous system. A B12 deficiency can manifest in mood swings, confusion, memory lapses, lack of appetite, vertigo, muscle weakness, or tingling sensations in the arms and legs. A prolonged deficiency can develop into hallucinations, paranoia, and mania. It does take a long time to become B12-deficient, though, since the body stores surpluses in the liver that can last about three to five years.

A deficiency is usually caused by a lack of intrinsic factor (IF), an enzyme (protein) that enables the absorption of vitamin B12 in the gut. Since levels of this enzyme drop with age, it's more common to encounter B12 deficiencies in older people. Vegetarians and vegans need to take extra B12, since their diets typically lack this vitamin. If you take contraceptive pills, breastfeed, or smoke cigarettes, you'll empty your body's reserves of B12 more quickly, and might also need to take a supplement.

Good sources of B vitamins are organic, grass-fed meat, fish, shellfish, milk, cheese, eggs, and liver, among other things.

Vitamin D is produced by the body when we're exposed to the sun. A lack of vitamin D can contribute to depression, while normal levels of vitamin D are good for mental health and mood. When the days become shorter and colder during winter, it is harder for the body to produce enough of it. People who live in colder climates, where the hours of sunlight are significantly less at certain times of the year, have a higher risk of becoming vitamin D–deficient, and they might experience seasonal depression. Taking a supplement during the darker months can help prevent this.

Additional research tells us that a vitamin D deficiency affects the immune system, and it is also suspected to be linked to a long list of illnesses, such as infectious diseases, cancer, cardiovascular disease, osteoporosis, generalized pain/fibromyalgia, and obesity.

A diet rich in vitamin D is a vital complement to the sun's UVB rays for people living in northern Europe and North America, especially during the darker season, from September to April. Levels of vitamin D (25-hydroxy vitamin D) can be easily checked with a blood test. Not all physicians and experts within the field agree on the best levels of vitamin D, but according to Sweden's Karolinska University laboratory, 30–100 ng/ml (75–250 nmol/l) is an optimal value.

Some good sources of vitamin D are fatty fish and enriched dairy products, and to a lesser extent organic, grass-fed meat and eggs.

SUGGESTION IF YOUR DIET LACKS ADEQUATE NUTRIENTS AND SUN-HOURS ARE FEW:
Vitamin D3
1,000–5,000 iu daily

"

A normal level of vitamin D is good for mental health and mood.

"

2. AVOID INFLAMMATION

Today, inflammation is suspected of being a strong contributing factor in many illnesses and health problems, such as cardiovascular disease, asthma, stroke, obesity, diabetes, dementia, depression, and cancer. But inflammation can cause imbalances in the hormone and neurotransmitter systems, too.

The immune system is one of the body's most critical systems. It prevents illnesses and promotes health and vitality. Inflammation is the immune system's first response to an acute infection and irritation, manifesting itself as swelling, redness, heat, and pain. Inflammation is important in quickly healing acute injuries like abrasions, a broken leg, or a wasp sting.

On the other hand, chronic inflammation that slowly simmers inside us can lead to problems. Over the long run, it can damage organs, threaten our health, cause imbalance in hormones and neurotransmitters, and hasten the aging process.

Treatments using anti-inflammatory medications like ibuprofen or acetylsalicylic acid, or steroids like cortisone, work well in acute injuries. However, if used over a long period, these medications can upset the body's immune system and cause serious side effects like gastritis, IBS (irritable bowel syndrome), IBD (irritable bowel disease), and leaky gut.

Unfortunately, within our health care system it's common to only treat the symptoms of inflammation without investigating its root cause. What we should do instead is identify what first brought this inflammation on. The reasons could be obesity, insulin resistance (see p. 32), GMOs (genetically modified organisms, such as corn, soy, or rapeseed), hidden food allergies, environmental allergens (chemical pesticides), stress, dental cavities, gingivitis, living a sedentary lifestyle, hidden infections due to parasites or an imbalance in gut flora, and of course certain foods in our diet (primarily those containing too much sugar).

Dairy products can also cause inflammation if you are lactose intolerant or allergic to milk. Goat, sheep's, and cow's milk contain varying amounts of fat, carbohydrates, and proteins. Cow's milk contains two proteins, casein (about 80 percent) and whey protein (about 20 percent), and the main carbohydrate in cow's milk is the milk sugar called lactose. You can be allergic to (or not be able to tolerate) casein, whey, or lactose. And if you can't tolerate either casein or whey itself, you

NEW SCIENTIFIC RESEARCH
Scientists at the Harvard School of Public Health have conducted a large study that, for the first time, shows a correlation between the Western world's inflammation-causing diets and our worsening mental health. Women who consumed large quantities of heavily sweetened drinks, refined white flour, red meat, and margarine ran a greater risk of suffering from depression, compared to those who ate a diet that was less inflammation-inducing.

won't be able to eat lactose-free dairy products since they still contain those ingredients.

A true milk *allergy* often causes rapid, acute reactions such as itching, swelling of the mouth and throat, or palpitations, while a food *intolerance* produces less acute but longer-lasting effects, with symptoms including stomachache, bloating, diarrhea, constipation, itching, and breakouts. However, new research shows that dairy products can actually inhibit inflammation in those who are not intolerant or allergic.

STRESS AND INFLAMMATION

Stress also increases the risk of inflammation in the body. When you're in a difficult situation, your nervous system reacts with a "fight or flight" response. The stress hormone cortisol is secreted, elevating levels of blood glucose, which gives your muscles quick energy and strength and allows you to defend yourself against sudden danger. If your day is full of stress from work, family, your finances, the Internet, or the constant aim for perfection, you increase your risk of having constantly high levels of cortisol and blood glucose in the body.

This in turn leads to hormonal disturbances, weight gain, insulin resistance, and diabetes, and over the long-term, inflammation in the body. Your good health and hormonal balance will depend on a lifestyle change and an anti-inflammatory diet.

To find out if you have inflammation, and the extent of it, you can request a C-reactive protein (CRP) blood test. This protein is produced by the liver in reaction to inflammation. A normal CRP should be less than 3 mg/l, while a higher reading indicates inflammation. Ask your physician to order the test if you want to rule out food allergies, food intolerances, parasites, and a lack of good gut bacteria. If your primary physician doesn't know about these tests, go to a clinic specializing in functional medicine.

INCREASE YOUR INTAKE OF ANTI-INFLAMMATORY FOOD

Anti-inflammatory food is packed with vitamins, antioxidants, and monounsaturated fats, and it contains only small amounts of sugar and polyunsaturated fats. Fill your plate with food containing organic protein like fish (opt for cold-water species like herring and salmon), fruit, nuts, vegetables, garlic, and spices such as turmeric, curry, and ginger.

HOW TO INFLUENCE INFLAMMATION FACTORS
· Reduce stress in your life.
· Visit your dentist regularly, and floss daily.
· Reduce your intake of sugar, refined white flour, and red meat.

3. BALANCE YOUR BLOOD GLUCOSE

The carbohydrates we eat are broken down into sugar (glucose), which is what the body and the brain use for quick energy. Certain carbohydrates provide longer-lasting mental and physical energy, while others cause hormonal disturbances, drops in blood glucose, fatigue, dizziness, and apathy.

Simple, fast-acting carbohydrates (in foods that are loaded with sugar, corn syrup, fruit juices, and refined wheat flour) are quickly converted to glucose, which rushes into the blood and spikes the blood sugar. If the body didn't have a way to lower this high level of blood glucose, we would eventually fall into a coma and die.

Fortunately, we've got our pancreas, which produces insulin. When blood glucose levels rise, more insulin is secreted to quickly force the excess glucose out of the bloodstream and into the cells. Insulin works like a key that opens the cells that are going to absorb the glucose; it simply unlocks the doors so the glucose can get in. Glucose is then used as fuel by the body.

However, if we have too much glucose, it will be stored as fat in different areas around the body. In women, it is often stashed in the bust and around the waistline, but also in the heart's coronary arteries. When your insulin level is high— if you eat too many fast-acting carbohydrates—it's pretty much impossible to lose weight. Over time this system can wear out—your insulin's effect weakens and the excess glucose will remain in the blood.

The condition in which insulin loses its effectiveness is called insulin resistance, which will increase the risk of inflammation in the body. Insulin resistance can block estrogen receptors, making it more difficult for estrogen to enter the cells.

Insulin can have a temporary effect on estrogen receptors, too. Here's an example: Let's say you're in menopause and you use hormone replacement therapy. You feel good and in balance—you sleep well, and your mood is even. One evening, during a dinner with some friends, you eat some bread, enjoy a very sweet dessert, and drink a few glasses of wine—all food and drink with a high carbohydrate content. As a result, your blood glucose and insulin levels spike. That night, you'll wake with hot flashes, unable to go back to sleep. The next day you'll be irritable and walk around in a fog. What happened? Well, you're suffering from a lack of estrogen because insulin is sitting in the estrogen receptors, blocking estrogen from entering the cells.

Insulin resistance increases the risk of hormonal disturbances with, among other things, an increased production of male sex hormones.

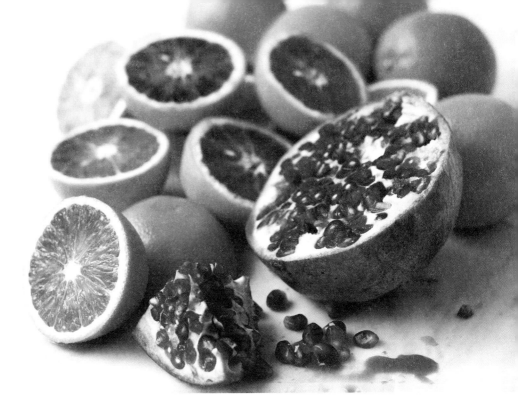

Insulin resistance raises the risk of hormonal disturbances due to an increased production of the male sex hormones DHEA (dehydroepiandrosterone) and testosterone, which causes increased hair growth or hirsutism (on the face and stomach and around the nipples), infertility, acne, and PCOS (polycystic ovary syndrome), a condition in which one or both ovaries are filled with small liquid-filled blisters called cysts, which can be seen by ultrasound.

OPT FOR SLOW-RELEASE CARBOHYDRATES!
Slow carbohydrates are full of fiber, vitamins, and minerals, which provide the brain and body with an even flow of glucose. This helps to maintain a sustained level of energy and normal hormone levels. With this comes a steadier and better mood. Slow carbohydrates can be found in nuts, beans, berries, fruits, vegetables, and legumes.

The recipes in this book feature wholesome carbohydrates that are broken down slowly in the stomach and the intestines, which result in hormonal balance, weight loss, and overall well-being.

4. KEEP YOUR GUT HAPPY

Good gut bacteria, or flora, enable the digestive system to break down food and reabsorb its nutrients.

The intestines, one of the largest organs in the body, are part of a delicate system that can become disrupted all too easily. Gut flora in the intestines play many important roles and is extremely complex and sensitive. It's made up of several billions of microorganisms that comprise over one thousand types of bacteria, weighing approximately 4½ lb (2 kg) together.

The number of "friendly" bacteria—the lactobacilli—decreases in our digestive system as we grow older, which is one of the reasons why older people are at greater risk for developing digestive issues like constipation and diarrhea.

LEAKY GUT SYNDROME

Digestive bacteria have more responsibilities than simply to break down food. In fact, bacteria are vital for your overall well-being. Unfortunately, lactobacilli are easily knocked out by stress hormones, toxins (poisons from both your food and environment), or antibiotics. Too few lactobacilli in the intestines affects the immune system, hormones, and body weight. It can lead to an increased permeability of the intestinal lining, what we call a leaky gut.

Leaky gut syndrome is when the typically strict regulation of what's being absorbed into the body through the intestinal mucosa and what goes out as fecal matter isn't working. Instead, bacteria, fungi, undigested particles of food, and other damaging substances can pass through the intestinal mucosa. The immune system becomes overactive and confused, and fires up an immune response that can attack its own body, nervous system, and joints.

This immune reaction can bring on fatigue, pain, osteoarthritis, food allergies, brain fog, asthma, and breakouts, as well as autoimmune diseases such as Hashimoto's thyroiditis (inflammation of the thyroid gland) and rheumatoid arthritis.

SUGGESTION IF YOUR DIET LACKS ADEQUATE NUTRIENTS:

Probiotics are supplements that contain healthy lactobacilli for gut flora. Try to find a supplement with high levels of bifidobacteria and lactobacilli (10–50 billion bacteria per capsule). There are even dairy-free probiotics available if you have lactose intolerance.

Another type of supplement is called prebiotics. Prebiotics are complex carbohydrates that are not broken down early in the digestive tract, but instead reach the colon in their original form. Prebiotics provide nourishment for the probiotic microorganisms and promote their growth. FOS (fructooligosaccharides) and inulin are the most common types of supplements.

DYSBIOSIS

Bifidobacteria and lactobacilli are key components to a healthy gut flora, while the bacteria enterococcus, streptococcus, and Escherichia coli (often shortened to E. coli), which also exist naturally in the body, can cause illness. It's easy to think that some bacteria are good and some are bad, but that would be wrong. In fact, the key factor here is maintaining a balance between the two. An imbalance in the gut between healthy and illness-causing bacteria is called dysbiosis, and it can have many different root causes, such as the consumption of improperly handled food, ingesting bacteria your body isn't accustomed to, or even taking a course of antibiotics.

Good bacteria play a vital role in regulating your hormones (especially estrogen). They help your body get rid of waste products from estrogen once it has been used. Naturally occurring estrogen, as well as any estrogen you have ingested via contraceptive pills or hormone replacement, must be broken down in the liver, moved out through the gallbladder to the small intestine and on to the colon, and out in the feces.

If you suffer from dysbiosis, the level of the enzyme in your colon, beta-glucuronidase, is often too high, which means that the broken-down hormones and toxins that are in the colon get reabsorbed into the body through the intestinal mucosa instead of being flushed out. This causes overly high levels of toxins and estrogen in the body. Adding probiotics to your diet can increase the good bacteria in your gut and regulate beta-glucuronidase levels.

More and more studies are showing that gut bacteria also affect body weight. In a study published in *Nature*, French scientists followed two groups over nine years, one made up of 169 overweight subjects, and the other of 123 subjects of regular weight. The group with individuals of regular weight had a larger number of healthy bacteria, as well as a much larger variety of bacteria, compared to the overweight people in the other group.

During my clinical practice, I often recommended my patients to do stool samples to check the balance of good and bad bacteria in the intestines. This is very common among practitioners practicing functional medicine.

> *Good gut bacteria play a vital role in regulating your hormones . . .*

COMMON SYMPTOMS OF DYSBIOSIS
- Bloating, belching, stomach catarrh, gas after meals
- Brain fog
- Acne
- Never feeling full or satiated
- Diarrhea and/or constipation
- Itchy skin, ears, anus
- Weak or split nails
- Iron deficiency
- Chronic fungal infections
- Fatigue
- Irregular or amenorrhea
- Swelling
- Tender breasts
- Weight gain

DYSBIOSIS AND ESTROGEN DOMINANCE

A deficiency in good gut bacteria over a long time can cause a slow buildup of estrogen in the body. If the level of progesterone is too low compared to estrogen, you will have what is called estrogen dominance.

Estrogen dominance can cause infertility, PMS, painful menstrual cramps, and heavy flow. It can also affect thyroid hormones, with a lowered metabolism and weight gain as a result. The imbalance between estrogen and progesterone also commonly leads to fluid buildup in the body. (Read more about estrogen dominance on p. 17.)

Also, ingest healthy, active bacteria via your diet by consuming fermented foods like sauerkraut, olives, pickled cucumbers, kimchi, yogurt, and kefir.

MODIFY YOUR DIETARY HABITS

As Westerners, we cannot maintain an environment of healthy gut flora if we don't make a conscious effort to change our dietary habits. The food we currently eat actively works against a balanced gut flora, and if we wish to keep ourselves hormonally balanced and at a healthy weight, we must create a conducive environment in our guts for lactobacilli to thrive.

So, how should you eat in order to protect these necessary, friendly bacteria? First, if possible, you should avoid taking antibiotics and decrease the amount of sugar and refined white flour in your diet. Eat more vegetables with high fiber content, such as onions, Jerusalem

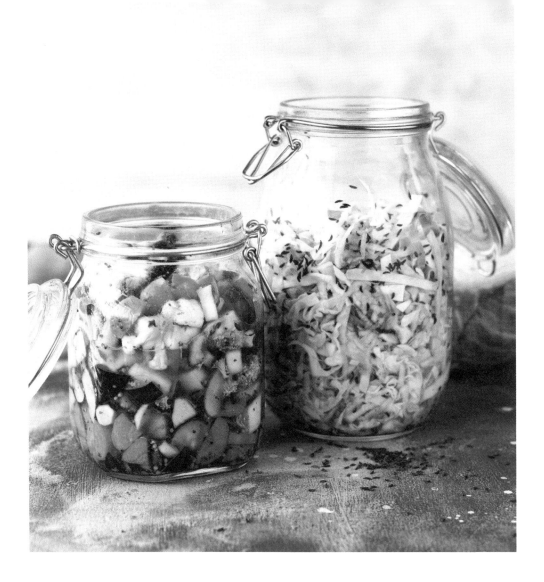

artichokes, starch-free root vegetables, green vegetables, apples, and legumes.

Also, ingest healthy, active bacteria via your diet by eating fermented foods like sauerkraut, olives, pickled cucumbers, kimchi, yogurt, and kefir.

Vegetables such as white cabbage, broccoli, Brussels sprouts, bok choy, and cauliflower also have a positive effect on the intestinal system, on health, and on estrogen dominance as they contain the substance indole-3-carbinol, which assists the liver in neutralizing toxic substances and ridding the body of used-up estrogen.

Fermented vegetables with turmeric, and sauerkraut with apple and cumin. Great for the lactobacilli in our intestines! Refer to the recipes on p. 112.

5. TRIM YOUR DIGESTION

For your body to absorb the nutrients in your food, digestive enzymes need to break down the food into small, separate molecules, which then pass through the intestinal wall and into the blood. Digestion begins in the mouth, so chew your food thoroughly.

Digestive enzymes are produced in the liver and in the pancreas. While there are many different types of enzymes, the most common of these are protease, lipase, and amylase. Protease breaks down proteins, lipase takes care of the fats, and amylase handles the carbohydrates. The production of enzymes decreases as we age, as well as in times of stress, and this leads to poor digestion and nutrient uptake.

To break down protein-rich foods, we also need gastric (hydrochloric) acid, which is produced in the stomach. It protects against bacteria, viruses, and parasites that you ingest every day by way of the food you eat and the liquids you drink. Hydrochloric acid also stimulates the secretion of the protein (enzyme) intrinsic factor (IF), which is necessary for the absorption of vitamin B12 and folic acid (B9). Gastric acid production, too, falls with age and increased levels of stress.

Common symptoms of enzyme deficiency are gas, belching, a bloated abdomen, and gastric reflux. If you suffer from any of these symptoms, try adding digestive enzymes to every meal to see if that will alleviate any problems. You shouldn't be feeling your food after you've eaten it, at least not until it's time to visit the bathroom.

Naturally occurring digestive enzymes can be found in different types of foods, for example fermented vegetables, papaya, pineapple, and mango.

A SIGN OF GOOD DIGESTION

You should have at least one good bowel movement per day, but two or three is optimal. A normal bowel movement is light brown in color, similar in consistency to toothpaste, and the size of a regular banana. Fecal matter is not supposed to float; floating feces can be a sign that your body is having trouble digesting and absorbing fats from the food (a high fat content in feces makes it float). Ideally, the time a meal takes to travel from mouth to toilet should be less than twenty-four hours.

> "
>
> *The digestion of food begins in the mouth, so chew thoroughly.*
>
> "

SUGGESTION IF YOUR DIET IS INADEQUATE: Take digestive enzymes with meals. There are many different supplements available on the market, but I recommend one that contains all three: amylase, lipase, and protease. Hydrochloric acid is also helpful at mealtimes: Betaine HCL, 500–1000 mg.

6. LOWER YOUR STRESS

Your ovaries produce the sex hormones estrogen, progesterone, and some testosterone; you need these hormones to feel healthy and well-balanced. However, the ovaries themselves don't know how much of the hormones to secrete into the body or when to secrete them. These responsibilities are driven entirely by the pituitary gland in the brain. I call the pituitary gland "the hormone conductor," because it acts like a conductor for the body's full hormonal orchestra.

The pituitary gland is a small gland that checks on hormone levels and ensures that the ovaries produce the right number of hormones at the right time, day and night, and at the correct time of the month. It's extremely sensitive to stress, and it notices if you're not eating well, if you're exercising too hard, or if you're tired or feeling ill. In the latter case, the pituitary gland makes sure you can't become pregnant by cutting off signals to the ovaries that would normally lead to the secretion of the hormones that trigger ovulation, which would typically provide hormonal balance. You can think of this gland as a protective mechanism for your body that ensures you don't get pregnant when your body isn't ready for it.

Starting today, try to do something that makes you happy.

WHAT MAKES YOU HAPPY?

While we're focusing on diet in this book, it's just as important to consider how you can lower stress in your life and become more present in the here and now. Be honest with yourself: how much time do you set aside to participate in things that mean a lot to you and that make you happy? Far too little, would be my guess. Women in their thirties to midfifties don't only go through hormonal changes; they are also often affected by significant amounts of external stress. Perhaps you see yourself trapped among difficult teenagers, aging parents, a strained marriage, and a stressful job. Most of us spend a lot of time taking care of others, rushing from one commitment to the next. We often find that we're unable to say "no" and make far too little time for ourselves.

Do you dream of taking a desert island vacation just to get away from all your to-do lists? You're not alone. But since this isn't financially realistic or practical for most of us, give some thought to how you can reduce stress in your everyday life, to avoid becoming exhausted or burned out.

I often urge my patients to stop for a moment and ask themselves, "What makes me happy?" Do you want to spend more time with your friends or your partner? Perhaps you'd like to enjoy a day at a spa, get a massage, go to the movies, or go on a nature hike. Maybe you just want to sleep. Whatever it is, it's very important that you give yourself permission to do it! Lower the bar and stop struggling to be perfect at everything you do. Step back, take a deep breath, and become aware of your own needs and what pleases you. Starting today, try to do something that makes you happy.

MEDITATION, YOGA, AND BREATHING

Meditation, yoga, and different breathing exercises are all excellent options for reducing stress. Even mindfulness—being present in the moment—is a good and practical way by which you can combat stress. CBT (cognitive behavioral therapy) can help you to analyze and work through your thoughts and behaviors, which in turn will show you the reasons you feel so stressed out. Once you know the source of your stress, it'll become much easier to deal with.

Since stress can lead to a deficiency in omega-3s and B vitamins (B6, folic acid [B9], and B12), I often recommend my patients who suffer from stress to take them as dietary supplements, even if they already eat a generally healthy diet.

Knowing the source of your stress makes it much easier to deal with.

BIOIDENTICAL HORMONES

We're focusing on diet in this book because it's the foundation of hormonal health. But as I've said, I also advocate for the use of bioidentical hormones. If you wish to take bioidentical hormones to achieve better balance in your body, you'll find plenty of advice and tips in my book *Female Brain Gone Insane* and on my website, mialundin.com.

What are bioidentical hormones, and in what ways are they different from synthetic hormones? Synthetic hormones are chemically altered molecules the body doesn't recognize, while bioidentical hormones have the same molecular structure as the body's own natural hormones. Because of this, the body recognizes bioidentical hormones and works with them in the same way it would with natural hormones produced by the ovaries. This returns an unwell body back to a balance and makes uncomfortable symptoms disappear.

Today, more and more scientific research is investigating the efficiency and safety of bioidentical hormones. Although the wheels of progress turn slowly at times, the advantages of bioidentical treatments have been demonstrated more and more, showing them as safe and effective methods for women seeking relief from perimenopausal and menopausal symptoms. Hormone experts all over the world agree that it is safe to use hormone treatments and that healthy women in the first ten years of menopause who need help alleviating their symptoms and preventing age-related disease need not be afraid to use hormone replacements.

Taking into consideration new scientific research, as well as my own twenty-five years or so of clinical experience, I have absolutely no doubt that a correct hormonal balance, by way of bioidentical hormones, keeps the mind focused, the body healthier, and the soul happier. Bioidentical hormones can minimize the risk of age-related illness since they keep levels of cholesterol and development of plaque in the arteries low. This in turn means a significant decrease in the likelihood of developing cardiovascular disease, without increasing the risk of getting breast cancer. Bioidentical hormones can only be obtained by prescription from a gynecologist or primary physician. (However, you can buy progesterone cream online.)

On the other hand, since synthetic hormones feature chemically manipulated molecules that are not recognized by our bodies, they can lead to undesirable side effects, such as nervousness, anxiety, and depression, and they increase the risk of developing blood clots and breast cancer.

Read more about bioidentical hormones in my book, Female Brain Gone Insane: An Emergency Guide for Women Who Feel That They Are Falling Apart, *and on my website,* mialundin.com.

BIOIDENTICAL ESTROGEN

Bioidentical estrogen is often derived from the soy plant. It is synthesized (altered) in a laboratory to arrive at the same exact molecular structure as the endogenous estrogen produced by the ovaries. Estradiol (17β -estradiol) is an example of bioidentical estrogen.

Today, most doctors prescribe bioidentical estrogens. A few examples that are available by prescription are Vivelle patch®, Divigel®, and Estrogel®. Several studies have shown that, contrary to earlier suspicions, transdermal estrogen (administered through the skin through a gel or patch) does not increase the risk of blood clots or stroke. A new Swedish study from 2015 confirms these findings.

BIOIDENTICAL PROGESTERONE

Progesterone is the first hormone that declines as we age. In our mid-to-late thirties, progesterone levels start to drop with the decline in ovulation. Low progesterone levels cause PMS and perimenopausal symptoms. Menopausal women who use estrogen and still have a uterus must also take a bioidentical progesterone, or synthetic progesterone (progestins), to prevent the development of cancer of the uterus. Many gynecologists and physicians still prescribe synthetic progesterone instead of bioidentical progesterone, even though several recent studies have shown that synthetic progesterone increases the risk of breast cancer. It is also very common for synthetic progesterone to cause anxiety, nervousness, and depression, while bioidentical progesterone is calming and very rarely causes any side effects.

HORMONE REPLACEMENT THERAPY

I'm often asked about the different types of hormone replacement therapies and about which products are bioidentical and which are synthetic. I've drawn up a list here so you can see which type of product you're using, or what you should ask for.

ESTROGEN, BIOIDENTICAL
Oral
Estrace® (1 mg and 2 mg estradiol)
Examples of Transdermal Estradiol

Name	Delivery method	Dosing
Vivelle Dot®	Transdermal patch	Twice weekly
EstroGel®	Topical gel	1–4 pumps daily
Divigel®	Transdermal gel	1 pack daily

Estrace vaginal cream® 0.01%
Vagifem, vaginal tablets 10 mcg

PROGESTERON, BIOIDENTICAL
Oral
Prometrium® 100 and 200 mg
Progesterone 100 and 200 mg

Vaginal
(used primarily for fertility treatment)
Prometrium 100 and 200 mg
Crinone Vaginal gel 8%

Cream
Progesterone cream * 20 mg per gram or
  pump. For treatment of PMS and
  perimenopause.

SYNTHETIC PROGESTERONE
(also called progestins)
Provera 5 and 10 mg (Medroxyprogesterone
  Acetate)
Mirena Intrauterine device (IUD),
  levonorgestrel, very low dosage progestin

COMBINED PREPARATIONS
(CONTAINS BIOIDENTICAL ESTROGEN AND
SYNTHETIC PROGESTERONE)
Oral

Activella	Estradiol/ Norethindrone Acetate	Pill
Angeliq	Estradiol/ Drospirenone	Pill
Femhrt	Norethindrone Acetate/ Ethinyl Estradiol	

Patch

Climara Pro	Estradiol/ Levonorgestrel	Patch
Combipatch	Estradiol/ Norethindrone Acetate	Patch

---

* Not recommended in combination with
estrogen during menopause, since there is no
research that shows progesterone cream can
prevent uterine cancer when used with estrogen. Can be purchased online.

SUMMARY, DIET LISTS, AND TABLES

Hopefully you now know a little more about food and different nutrients that favor your hormonal balance and your well-being. But maybe you're wondering about which ingredients you should eat and which ones you should avoid?

There is no special hormone diet; a diet for optimal hormonal balance is made up of a combination of different diets, such as the Mediterranean diet and the glycemic index diet, along with foods that promote healthy gut bacteria that reduce inflammation, insulin resistance, and weight gain.

By taking dietary advice and using the recipes from this book, you will hopefully enjoy life more, feel focused, have additional energy and harmony, and maybe even lose a bit of weight as a bonus!

PRACTICAL DIET TIPS—A SUMMARY
- Eat a varied diet containing animal protein—preferably fatty fish—several times a week. Eat plenty of vegetables, some fruit, and very few grains—choose gluten-free products or oats whenever possible.
- Eat organic protein during each main meal.
- Eat slow-release carbohydrates such as fruits, legumes, and vegetables.

INCLUDE THESE FOODS IN YOUR DIET
Organic meat: poultry (like turkey and chicken), veal, lamb, and game. Vegetable protein: lentils, quinoa, peanut butter, hemp protein powder, chia seeds, and almond milk. Legumes such as lentils, chickpeas, Borlotti beans, white beans, and kidney beans.

Fatty fish: mackerel, herring, salmon, char, and sardines. They contain lots of protein and wholesome fatty acids, and certain minerals.

Shellfish: shrimp, crawfish, crab, lobster, oysters, and mussels.

Vegetables: many, and a wide variety of them! Look for kale, white cabbage, Brussels sprouts, cauliflower, broccoli, and bok choy. These vegetables contain the substance indole-3-carbinol, which helps the liver neutralize toxins, and helps the body get rid of the estrogen that has been spent (estrogen metabolism).

Good fats: nuts, olives, avocado, extra virgin olive oil (omega-6), flaxseed oil (omega-3), coconut oil, and sesame seed oil. Good fats can also be found in cold-water fish like salmon, brown trout, char, and mackerel.

Fruit: 1 to 2 per day. Choose those that have the least effect on blood glucose, namely apples, pears, and oranges. But you can also opt for papaya, mango, and pineapple, which all contain substances that aid digestion.

Berries low on the glycemic index and full of Vitamin C: blueberries, raspberries, cherries, and rose hips.

Almond or oat milk as an alternative to regular dairy if you can't digest or are allergic to cow's milk.

Fermented foods: fermented vegetables, sauerkraut, olives, pickled brined cucumber, and kimchi.

Anti-inflammatory spices: turmeric, curry, and ginger.

Nuts: All nuts are healthy. Try new varieties! Different nuts contain different nutrients that are good for you. You have omega-3 in walnuts, for example, and selenium in Brazil nuts.

AVOID THESE FOODS

It's vital to provide your body with all the necessary nutrients it needs to produce hormones and neurotransmitters. But it's almost as important to reduce the intake of foods that can cause inflammation and allergies, because they too can affect your overall health and well-being.

- sugar
- gluten
- corn
- tomatoes (with diagnosed allergy or inflammation in the body)
- eggplant
- sunflower oil
- corn oil

Dairy products: Avoid them if you know that you can't tolerate or have an allergy to them, because they can cause inflammation in the body. On the other hand, if you can digest cow's milk or have no allergies, dairy products won't bring on inflammation.

Foods that lead to unstable blood glucose levels and an elevated insulin response: sugar, sodas, gluten, and fruit juices. If you want to sweeten your food, choose a sweetener like organic honey that hasn't been heated, agave syrup, or coconut sugar.

Alcohol: Although small amounts of red wine can help reduce the risk of cardiovascular disease, it still has no positive effect whatsoever on hormones and mood. Instead, alcohol blocks the estrogen receptors in the body and elevates the insulin response.

Certain artificial colorants (commonly found in sodas and candy): They can lead to hyperactivity, trouble concentrating, and lack of impulse control.

Artificial sweeteners: Aspartame is a common artificial sweetener used in, among other things, diet sodas and most brands of chewing gum. It contains chemical toxins that can disturb your neurotransmitters' function and cause migraines, depression, rage-like episodes, joint aches, and muscle spasms. It can also cause symptoms akin to multiple sclerosis, chronic fatigue syndrome, and fibromyalgia.

Trans-fatty acids (transfats): You'll find them in many processed foods, such as French fries, margarine, chips, biscuits, cookies, instant sauces, instant soups, ice cream, baking chocolate, bread, pastries, ready-to-eat meals, Fritos, stock cubes, and Promise® low-fat butter substitute.

IBD STUDY

A study published in the IBD Journal showed that inflammatory bowel disease could be caused by the artificial sweeteners saccharine and sucralose (Splenda®). These two sweeteners are common ingredients in today's light and diet products.

EXAMPLES OF INGREDIENTS FOR HORMONAL BALANCE

FATS AND OILS
avocado oil
fish oil
hazelnut (filbert) oil
peanut butter
coconut oil
olive oil
almond oil
almond butter
rapeseed oil

PROTEINS
Borlotti beans
chia seeds
organic pork and beef
hemp seeds
peanut butter
turkey
chickpeas
chicken
salmon
almond milk
char
herring
cod
white beans
eggs

VITAMIN C
pineapple
oranges
blueberries
pomegranate
grapefruit
raspberries
mango
blackberries
papaya
pears
apples

VEGETABLES AND ROOT VEGETABLES
avocado
cauliflower
broccoli
Brussels sprouts
kale
ginger
Jerusalem artichoke
onion
carrots
bok choy
parsnip
bell pepper
asparagus
spinach
sweet potatoes/yams
white cabbage
garlic
zucchini/summer
  squash

GRAINS AND SEEDS
chia seeds
hemp seeds
flaxseeds
groats (hulled oats)
quinoa
sunflower seeds

OMEGA-3
chia seeds
organic meat from
  grass-fed animals
  (or game)
cold-pressed flax oil
salmon, preferably
  wild-caught
flaxseeds
mackerel
omega-3 eggs
herring

MAGNESIUM
green leafy
  vegetables
beans
seeds
whole grain products
nuts

ZINC
whole grain products
chicken
nuts
shellfish

SELENIUM
algae
fatty fish
offal
meat
nuts
shellfish
eggs

IRON
organic meat
green peas
kale
leeks
sardines
spinach
egg yolk

VITAMIN B
fish
meat
liver
milk
cheese
shellfish
eggs

ANTI-INFLAMMATORY SEASONINGS
cayenne pepper
chili powder
lemon
curry
turmeric
ginger
red pepper

FIBER
legumes
oats
carrots
psyllium seeds
psyllium husk
apples

PROTEIN POWDERS
pea
hemp

NUTRITIONAL DEFICIENCIES AND THEIR SYMPTOMS

Vitamins and minerals are the facilitators, i.e., the enzymes that make practically every biochemical process in your body happen. Your health, mood, and behavior can suffer if you don't have enough of them.

I've used the table below in my clinical practice for many years. Here you can see the common symptoms for certain nutritional deficiencies, how common these deficiencies are, and a selection of raw ingredients where you can find the missing nutrients. If you think you might be suffering from a deficiency, first try eating more of the foods that contain the nutrient you're lacking. If this doesn't make you feel better, then try adding a dietary supplement to see if it will alleviate the symptoms.

NUTRIENT	HOW COMMON IS THIS NUTRIENT DEFICIENCY?	RAW INGREDIENT CONTAINING NUTRIENT	SYMPTOMS AND PROBLEMS CAUSED BY DEFICIENCY
Vitamin B1	Uncommon	Pork, liver, whole grain products, brown rice, brewer's yeast, molasses	Cognitive impairment, Alzheimer's disease
Vitamin B12	Very common	Brewer's yeast, almonds, liver, whole grain, mushrooms, soy, dairy products, eggs, dark green leafy vegetables	Anemia, cataracts, impaired thyroid function, B6 deficiency, fatigue
Vitamin B3	Uncommon	Beets, brewer's yeast, red meat, chicken, liver, fish, grains, nuts	Cracking and flaking skin, stomach/digestive problems, confusion, anxiety, fatigue
Vitamin B5	Uncommon	Red meat, vegetables, lentils, egg yolks, milk, whole grain products, beans, seeds, salmon	Skin problems, impaired stress tolerance, fatigue
Vitamin B6	Common	Chicken, tuna, salmon, shrimp, liver, lentils, seeds, nuts, avocado, bananas, carrots, brown rice, whole grains	Depression, anxiety, sleep disturbance, confusion, skin problems
Folic acid (B9)	Very common	Beans, lentils, dark green leafy vegetables, whole grain products, raspberries	Anemia, impaired immune function, fatigue, difficulty falling asleep, hair loss

NUTRIENT	HOW COMMON IS THIS NUTRIENT DEFICIENCY?	RAW INGREDIENT CONTAINING NUTRIENT	SYMPTOMS AND PROBLEMS CAUSED BY DEFICIENCY
Vitamin A	Uncommon	Milk, eggs, liver, oranges, dark green leafy vegetables, fruit	Night blindness, impaired immune system, zinc deficiency, impaired fat assimilation
Vitamin C	Common	Rose hips, guava, parsley, bell pepper, nettles, black currants, oranges	Bleeding gums, impaired wound healing; serious deficiency can cause scurvy
Vitamin D	Very common	Sunshine, milk, egg yolks, liver, fish	Fatigue, depression, muscle weakness, joint, muscle and skeletal pain, muscle cramps, difficulty getting up and walking up stairs
Vitamin K	Uncommon	Kale, green tea, turnips, spinach, lettuce, cabbage, beef liver, asparagus, cheese, oats, peas, whole grains	Serious bleeding, bruises, heavy menstrual flow
Vitamin E	Very common	Wheat germ, liver, eggs, seeds, cold-pressed vegetable oils, dark green leafy vegetables, avocado, asparagus, Brazil nuts	Skin and hair problems, bruising, PMS, hot flashes, eczema
Calcium	Very common	Dairy products, wheat, brewer's yeast, whole grains, sardines, salmon, cabbage, dark green leafy vegetables	Anxiety, muscle cramps, osteoporosis, irritability
Selenium	Common	Wheat germ, liver, butter, cold-water fish, shellfish, garlic, sunflower seeds, Brazil nuts	Dementia, high blood pressure, impotence, cataracts, skin problems, impaired thyroid function
Copper	Uncommon	Oysters, seeds, whole-grain bread, nuts, dark chocolate, shellfish, dark green leafy vegetables	Impaired immune system, osteoporosis, general weakness, impaired lung function, anemia, decreased pigmentation
Zinc	Very common	Oysters, red meat, chicken, beans, nuts, shellfish, dairy products	Hair loss, diarrhea, impotence, eye and skin irritations, loss of appetite, fatigue

RECIPES: FOOD THAT IS GOOD FOR YOU AND YOUR HORMONES

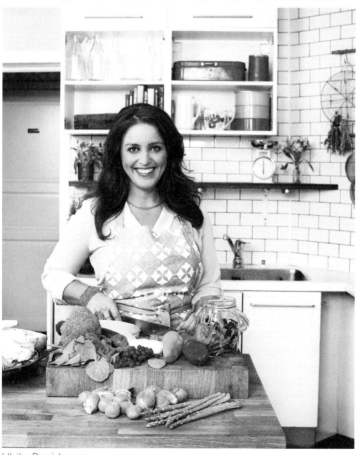

Ulrika Davidsson

To modify your lifestyle and the food you eat, you need to be willing to make some changes, now and over the long haul, and to do so with joy. Mia has helped you out with the facts, and now I'll share some simple and hormone-friendly recipes for fun and delicious dishes!

I hope the pictures will encourage you to move into the kitchen. Try out the dishes that look good to you and arouse your curiosity. Then, it's just a matter of gathering the ingredients and following the recipes; it doesn't get much simpler than that! If you don't like or can't eat a certain ingredient, you can easily replace it with something else.

The dishes center on natural proteins and fats and feature many vegetables, fruits, and berries. You'll steer clear of gluten and different grains as much as possible, so your carbohydrates will come from gluten-free sources like rice, quinoa, oats, lentils, beans, and root vegetables.

You'll enjoy new breakfast recipes for porridge, green smoothies, energy-rich smoothie bowls, and easy-to-bake gluten-free breads. Many of the lunches and dinners are relatively quick to make and will please everyone in the family. Prepare extra servings to enjoy for lunch the next day or store some in the freezer for later, when time is short or no one feels like cooking.

Since the recipes are low in carbohydrates, you'll notice that you'll feel full quickly. Most important, you'll lose your cravings for other foods and sweets. And if you'd like to spice up your week with a coffee break or a dessert, just bake a chocolate cake or make one of the other wholesome treats in this book. Whenever I eat good food like this, my entire body feels healthy and well.

I hope to inspire you to begin preparing these recipes! (You'll understand what I mean once you've followed the meal plan on p. 157.) The energy and time you devote to food will be rewarded with wonderful hormonal balance and overall health and well-being.

Here's wishing you a happy food experience!

Since the recipes are low in carbohydrates, you'll notice that you'll feel full quickly. Most important, you'll lose your cravings for other foods and sweets.

BREAKFASTS

It's good to start the day off by drinking plenty of water, preferably with some freshly squeezed lemon juice added in. Or why not down a shot of ginger and lime? It's a good cleanser first thing in the morning—it neutralizes your pH and boosts your immune defense. Choose one of your favorite breakfasts—try chia seeds, fruit and berries, rolled oats, or an omelet—and enjoy a relaxed and pleasant start to your day.

Ginger and lime shot 54 * Lemon water 55 * Chia porridge with mango and orange 57 * Chia porridge with chocolate crème 58 * Oatmeal "to go" 61 * Crunchy granola 62 * Green smoothie with basil 64 * Cottage cheese "to go" 65 * Yellow smoothie bowl 66 * Red smoothie bowl 66 * Scrambled eggs with brie cheese 69 * Omelet with pear, feta, and raspberries 70 * Flaxseed buns with cranberries 73 * "Faux" rye bread with flax and sunflower seeds 74

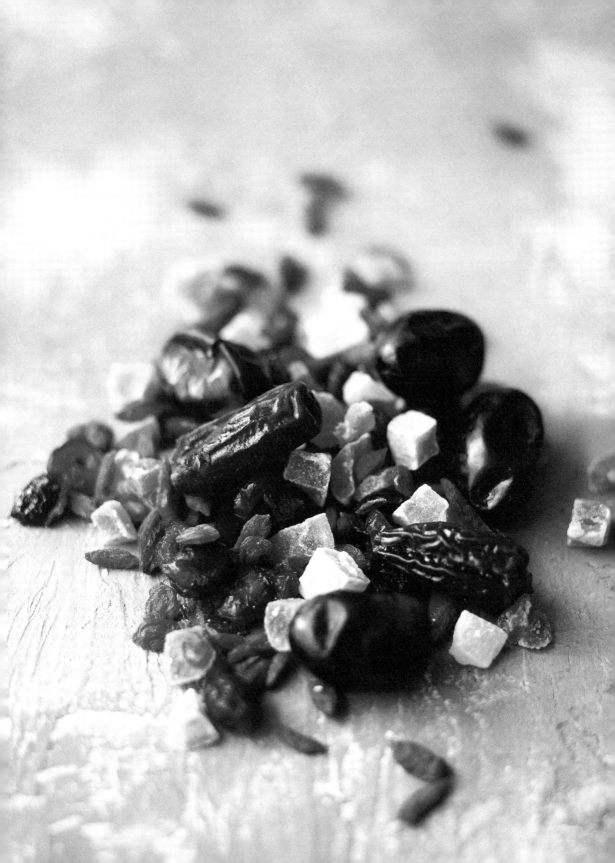

GINGER AND LIME SHOT

SERVES 1

Juice from 1 lime

1¼ cups (300 ml) cold water

1 tsp finely grated fresh
   ginger

1 tsp liquid honey

Mix lime juice, water, ginger, and honey in large glass or small pitcher. Stir until the honey has dissolved, and drink immediately in the morning.

By all means, start your morning off with a shot of ginger and lime or a glass of lemon water.

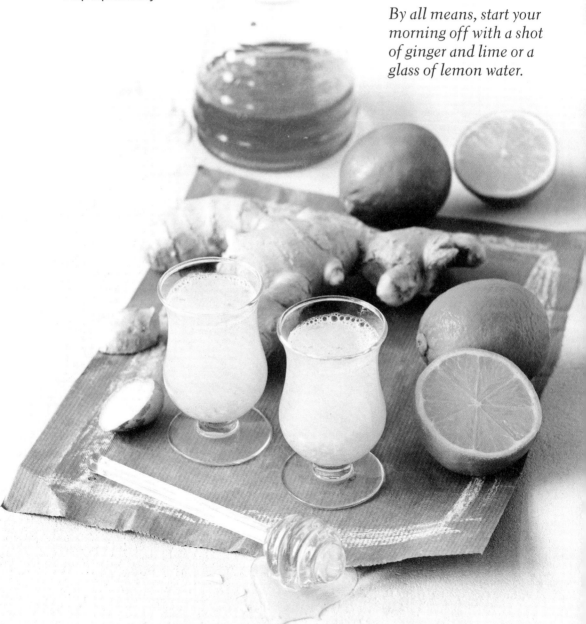

LEMON WATER

SERVES 1

Juice of ½ lemon, plus zest

2½ cups cold water

A few ice cubes

Grate some lemon zest into a glass pitcher, along with squeezed lemon juice. Add the water and ice, and stir. Drink the water in the morning.

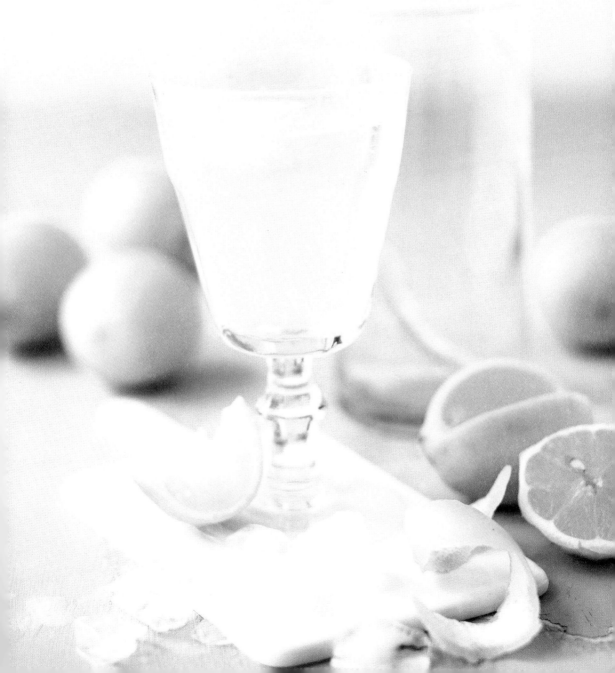

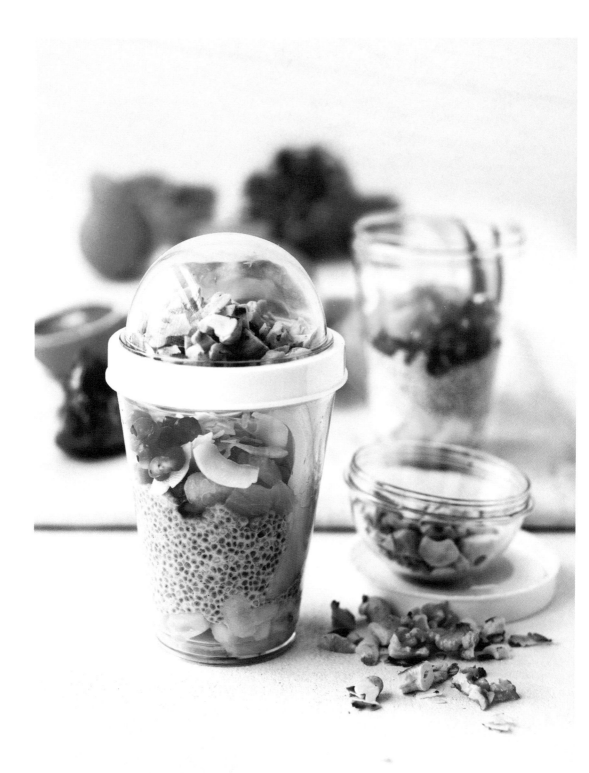

It's best to prepare the porridge in the evening and let it sit overnight in the refrigerator. Add the topping in the morning, and enjoy.

CHIA PORRIDGE WITH MANGO AND ORANGE

SERVES 2

4 tbsp chia seeds

1¼ cups oat milk

1 tsp liquid honey

⅖ cup (100 ml) frozen or fresh diced mango

TOPPING

1 orange

Seeds from ½ pomegranate

2 tbsp coconut chips

⅕ cup (50 ml) mixed nuts

1 tsp liquid honey

Stir the chia seeds, oat milk, and honey together in a bowl. Let the mixture sit overnight in the refrigerator, or for at least 2 hours.

If needed, defrost the diced mango and place in a serving bowl or jar. Top with the chia porridge.

Peel the orange and cut away the segments from the pith. Place the segments on the porridge along with the pomegranate seeds and coconut chips.

Toast the nuts in a dry skillet; add the liquid honey and mix. Coarsely chop the nuts, add them to the porridge, and serve.

CHIA PORRIDGE WITH CHOCOLATE CRÈME

4 tbsp chia seeds

1⅖ cups (300 ml) almond milk

1 tsp liquid honey

⅖ cup (100 ml) frozen raspberries

CHOCOLATE CRÈME

3 dried, pitted dates

1 tbsp cocoa

½ avocado

1 frozen, sliced banana

ACCOMPANIMENTS

⅕ cup (50 ml) fresh or frozen raspberries

1 banana, sliced

Stir the chia seeds, almond milk, honey, and frozen raspberries together in a bowl. Let the mixture sit in the refrigerator overnight, or for at least 2 hours.

Mix all ingredients for the chocolate crème until smooth.

Place some raspberries at the bottom of a glass or bowl. Layer with banana, porridge, and chocolate crème, and add more raspberries on top.

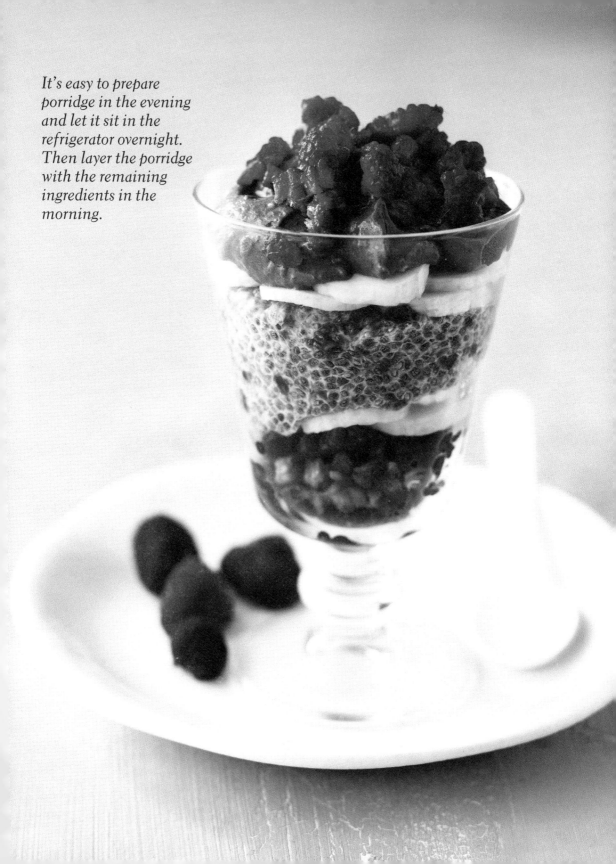

It's easy to prepare porridge in the evening and let it sit in the refrigerator overnight. Then layer the porridge with the remaining ingredients in the morning.

Fill a glass jar with rolled oats and your choice of flavoring. Let it sit in the refrigerator until you're off to work or away on a trip. When it's time to eat, just add boiling water and let it stand for 10 minutes. You'll have freshly made, very tasty porridge in a jiffy!

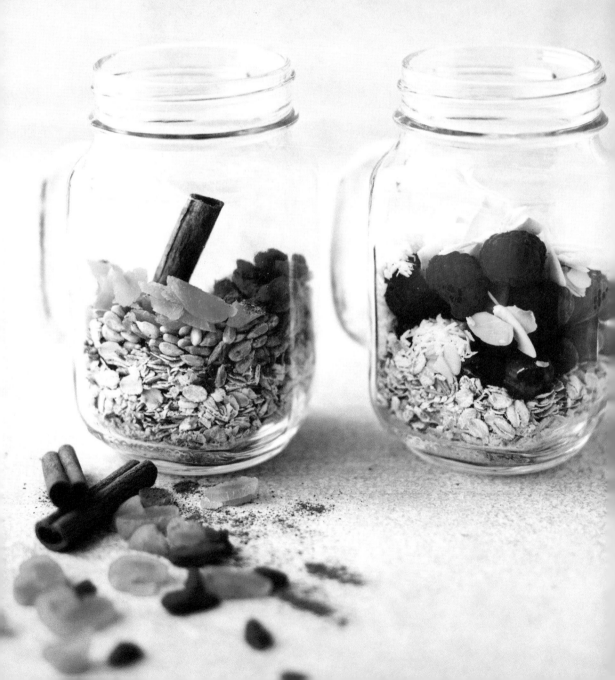

OAT PORRIDGE "TO GO"

SERVES 1

PORRIDGE WITH CINNAMON AND APRICOTS

- ⅔ cup (100 ml) rolled oats
- 1 tsp liquid honey
- 1 tbsp flaxseeds
- 2 tbsp sunflower seeds
- ⅓ tsp ground cinnamon
- ⅓ tsp ground cardamom
- 3 dried apricots, chopped
- 1 tbsp goji berries
- 1 stick cinnamon
- A pinch of salt
- ⅘ cup (200 ml) boiling water
- Oat or almond milk, for serving

SERVES 1

PORRIDGE WITH BERRIES AND COCONUT

- ⅔ cup (100 ml) rolled oats
- ⅓ tsp vanilla powder
- 1 tsp liquid honey
- 1 tbsp coconut flakes
- 2 tbsp almond flakes
- 2 tbsp coconut chips
- ⅕ cup (50 ml) fresh or frozen berries
- A pinch of salt
- ⅘ cup (200 ml) boiling water
- Oat or almond milk, for serving

Place all the ingredients (except water and milk for serving) in a glass jar and close with a lid. Store in the refrigerator.

Add the water and stir thoroughly. Put the lid back on again and let it sit for 10 minutes. Stir again and serve with oat or almond milk.

CRUNCHY GRANOLA

1⅔ cups (400 ml) rolled oats

⅘ cup (200 ml) almond flour

⅕ cup (50 ml) flaxseeds

⅕ cup (50 ml) sesame seeds

⅖ cup (100 ml) sunflower seeds

⅖ cup (100 ml) walnuts, coarsely chopped

1 tsp ground cinnamon

1 tbsp ground cardamom

3 tbsps coconut fat

2 tbsps liquid honey

3 tbsps water

⅖ cup (100 ml) coconut flakes

⅖ cup (100 ml) dried apricots, chopped, or golden raisins

⅖ cup (100 ml) goji berries

Preheat the oven to 400°F (200°C). Combine the rolled oats, almond flour, flaxseeds, sesame seeds, sunflower seeds, walnuts, cinnamon, and cardamom in a bowl. Melt the coconut fat in a saucepan, and drizzle it into the bowl along with the honey and water. Mix thoroughly.

Roast the mixture on a baking tray in the oven for 20 minutes. Stir a few times to make sure the granola doesn't burn. Remove the tray from the oven and add in the coconut, apricots, and goji berries. Let cool completely, and store in a jar with a tight-fitting lid.

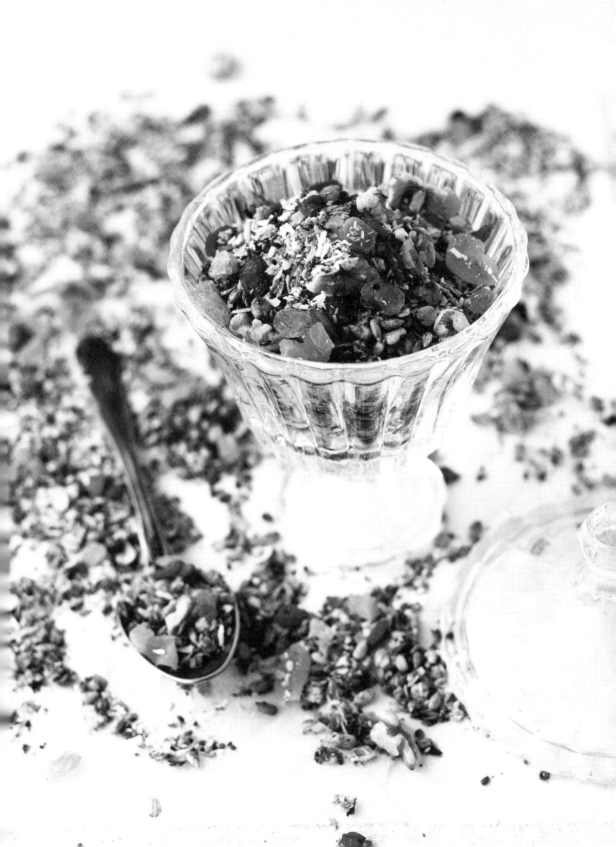

GREEN SMOOTHIE WITH BASIL

SERVES 2

½ fresh pineapple

½ bunch basil

1 oz (30 g) fresh spinach

Juice from ½ lime

⅕ cup (50 ml) water

Fresh raspberries for garnish
  (optional)

Peel the pineapple and cut it into chunks. Put the chunks in a food processor or a blender. Add the basil, spinach, and lime juice. Process to make a smoothie, and dilute with a little water. Pour into glasses and, if you like, garnish with some raspberries.

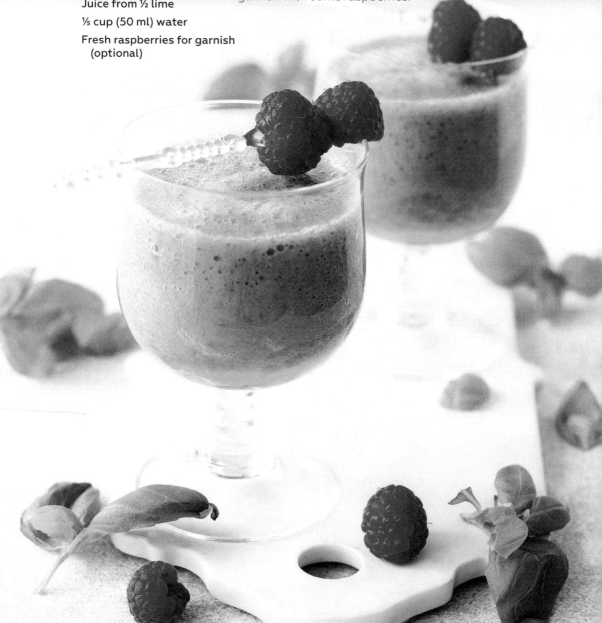

COTTAGE CHEESE "TO GO"

SERVES 2

⅕ cup (50 ml) fresh blueberries

4½ oz (125 g) 4% cottage cheese

Seeds from ½ pomegranate

⅕ cup (50 ml) diced fresh pineapple

1 kiwi, peeled and sliced

7 fresh raspberries

CRUNCHY TOPPING

Nut mix with ground cherries, cranberries, dried cherries, pumpkin seeds, and goji berries (can be store-bought and ready-to-eat)

Layer blueberries, cottage cheese, pomegranate seeds, pineapple, and kiwi in a bowl or cup. Garnish with raspberries. Sprinkle with some crunchy topping before eating.

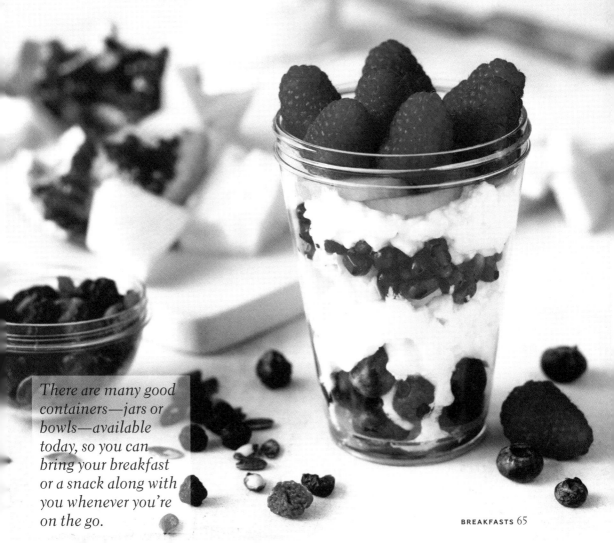

There are many good containers—jars or bowls—available today, so you can bring your breakfast or a snack along with you whenever you're on the go.

A satisfying and naturally fresh breakfast that you can prepare the night before, and bring out in the morning.

YELLOW SMOOTHIE BOWL

SERVES 1

¾ fresh pineapple

⅖ cup (100 ml) frozen, diced mango

1 banana

5 ground cherries

TOPPING

8 fresh raspberries, 2 tbsp pumpkin seeds, seeds from ½ pomegranate, seeds from ½ passion fruit, sliced star fruit

Place all the ingredients in a blender or food processor, and blend to a lump-free smoothie. Transfer the smoothie to a bowl, and garnish with the topping ingredients.

RED SMOOTHIE BOWL

SERVES 1

⅓ cup (75 ml) frozen blueberries

⅕ cup (50 ml) frozen raspberries

⅖ cup (100 ml) coconut cream

1 banana

TOPPING

⅕ cup (50 ml) fresh blueberries, ½ kiwi, 1 tbsp coconut flakes, 1 tsp hemp seeds, 4 ground cherries, ¼ nectarine

Place all the ingredients in a blender or food processor, and blend to a lump-free smoothie. Transfer the smoothie to a bowl, and garnish with the topping ingredients.

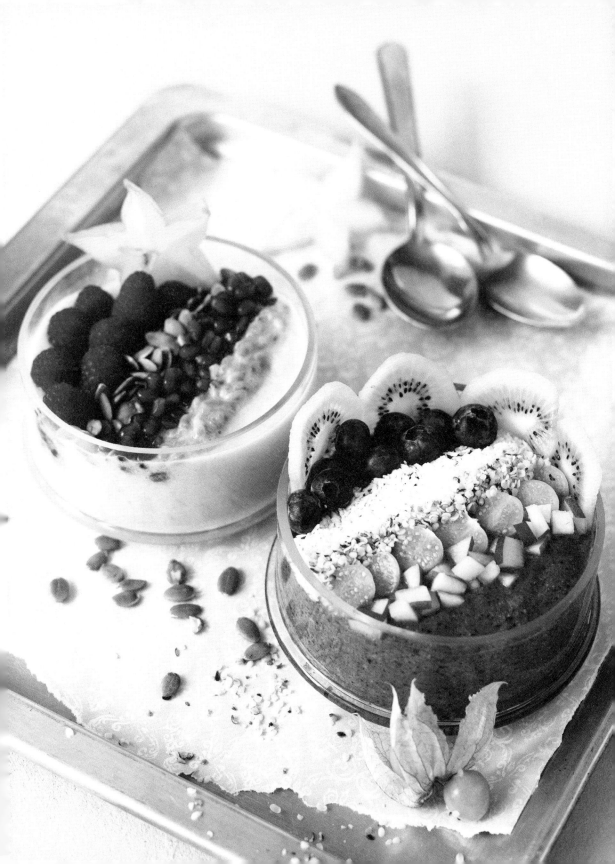

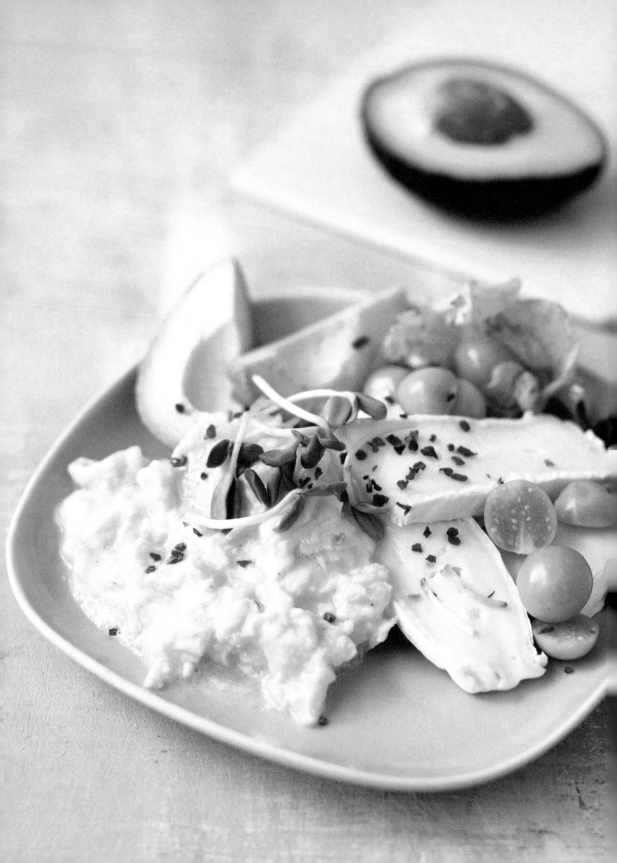

Scrambled eggs—a delicacy that is quickly put together and perfect for when you're hungry but short on time. By all means, feel free to use a variety of different cheeses and vegetables here.

SCRAMBLED EGGS WITH BRIE CHEESE

SERVES 1

2 eggs

Salt and white pepper

1 tsp butter

1 oz (30 g) brie, sliced

½ avocado

5 ground cherries

Green lettuce leaves

Sunflower sprouts or sandwich cress

Paprika and dried or fresh herbs, for sprinkling (optional)

Whisk together the eggs with salt and pepper in a bowl. Heat the butter in a skillet, and pour in the egg mixture. Stir for about 30 seconds, and then transfer the eggs to a plate. Top them with slices of brie, avocado, ground cherries, and lettuce leaves. Sprinkle with sunflower sprouts and optional herbs.

A winning combo for topping an omelet: pear, feta cheese, and raspberries.

OMELET WITH PEAR, FETA, AND RASPBERRIES

SERVES 1

2 eggs

Salt and white pepper

1 tsp butter

1 oz (30 g) feta cheese

½ pear, sliced

7 fresh raspberries

1 tsp almond flakes, toasted

Snipped cress, for garnish

Whisk together the eggs with salt and pepper in a bowl. Heat the butter in a skillet, and fry the omelet for a minute or two. Crumble some feta cheese over the eggs, and set the pear slices, raspberries, almond flakes, and cress on top.

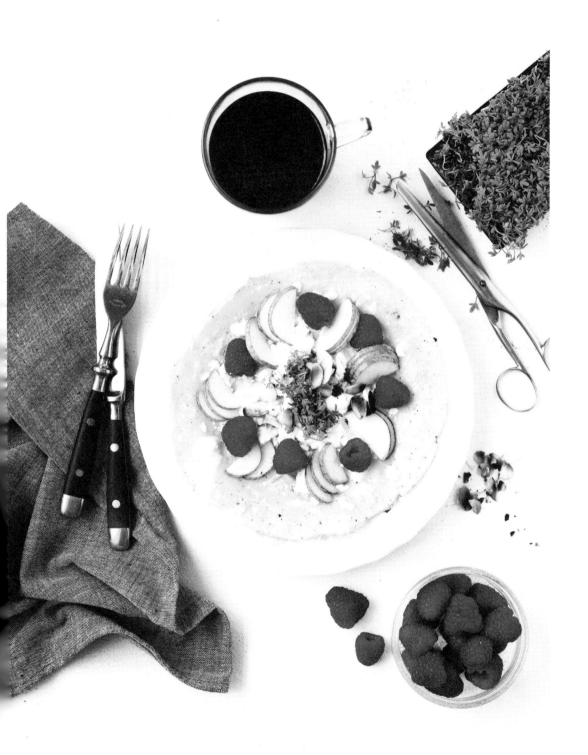

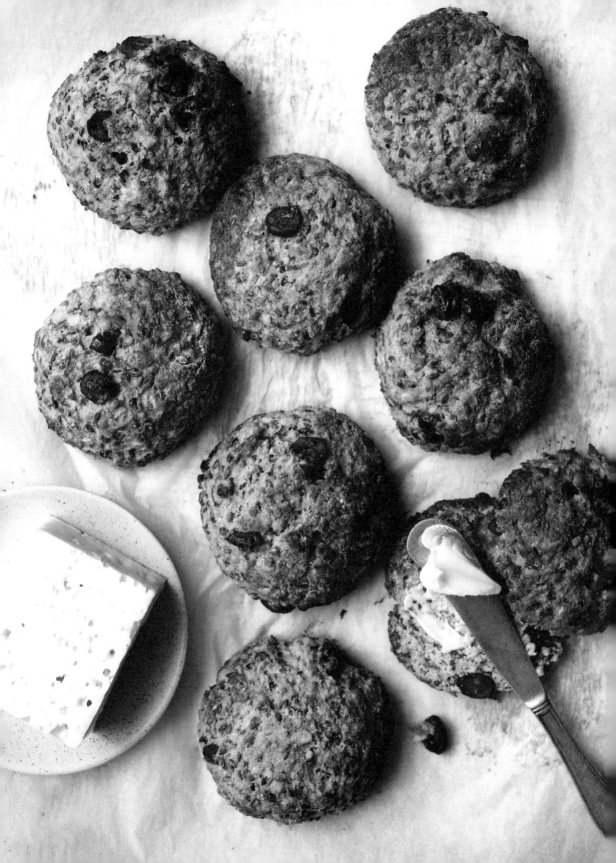

Bake and freeze. They're delicious when reheated in the oven or toasted!

FLAXSEED BUNS WITH CRANBERRIES

MAKES 8 BUNS

- 1 oz (25 g) fresh yeast (or equivalent amount in dried yeast)
- 2 cups cold milk
- 1 oz (25 g) rapeseed oil
- ⅓ oz (10 g) oat fiber
- 3½ oz (100 g) rolled oats
- 2½ oz (70 g) buckwheat
- 1 oz (25 g) soy flour
- ¾ oz (20 g) psyllium husk
- ⅛ tsp bread spices*
- ½ tsp salt
- ⅔ cup (100 ml) dried cranberries

Crumble the yeast into a bowl (or follow instructions on the packet of dried yeast). Add the milk and stir until the yeast has dissolved. Add the rest of the ingredients and mix to a smooth dough. Cover the bowl with plastic wrap, and let the dough rise for about 2 hours.

Preheat the oven to 437°F (225°C). Shape 8 buns and set them on a baking sheet covered with parchment paper. Bake on the middle rack of the oven for about 20 minutes, and then let the buns cool on a rack.

*Combine equal parts ground fennel, anise seeds, and caraway seeds, and grind to mix in a coffee grinder.

Wonderfully tasty gluten-free bread! It's easy to bake and stays fresh for up to five days.

"FAUX" RYE WITH FLAX AND SUNFLOWER SEEDS

MAKES 1 LOAF

2½ cups (600 ml) cultured milk or buttermilk

⅖ cup (100 ml) dark syrup

1½ cups (375 ml) buckwheat flour

⅓ cup (75 ml) soy flour

⅕ cup (50 ml) rose hip husk flour

⅖ cup (100 ml) flaxseeds

⅘ cup (200 ml) sunflower seeds

4 tbsp psyllium husks

1 tsp baking soda

FOR THE BAKING PAN

1 tsp butter, for greasing

1 tsp buckwheat flour

Preheat the oven to 350°F (175°C). Mix all the ingredients together in a bowl. Let the mixture rest and rise for a few minutes. Grease and flour a 1½–2 quart baking pan.

Transfer the dough evenly to the pan and sprinkle some buckwheat flour over the surface. Bake on the lower rack of the oven for about 50 minutes. Let it cool on a rack.

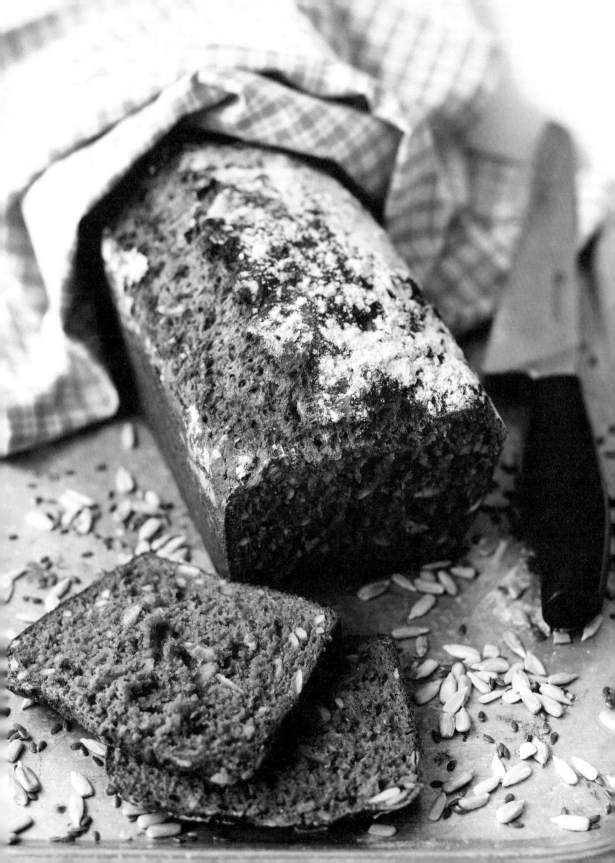

SALADS AND WARM SOUPS

"Salads in a jar" are a great invention. Just put different vegetables in a glass jar and bring it to work. Pour in some dressing, mix, and it's ready! I add a lot of raw vegetables to maximize the number of digestive enzymes, antioxidants, and nutrients.

Soup can be varied in a multitude of ways. Make a double batch and store it in the refrigerator—it's the ultimate fast food!

Zucchini pasta with pesto 78 * Melon salad with chèvre and avocado 81 * Mozzarella salad with Chioggia beets 82 * Marinated beets with chèvre gratin 85 * Chicken wrapped in rice paper 86 * Pear and blue cheese salad 88 * Asian salad 90 * Swedish salad 93 * Italian salad 94 * Arabian salad 97 * Raw food salad 98 * Mediterranean salad 101 * Omelet wrap with a selection of fillings 102 * Carrot soup with ginger and chicken bacon 105 * Spinach soup with avocado and green peas 107 * Tomato soup with halloumi cheese 108 * Asian salmon soup with seagrass noodles 110 * Fermented vegetables with turmeric 112 * Sauerkraut with apple and caraway seed 112

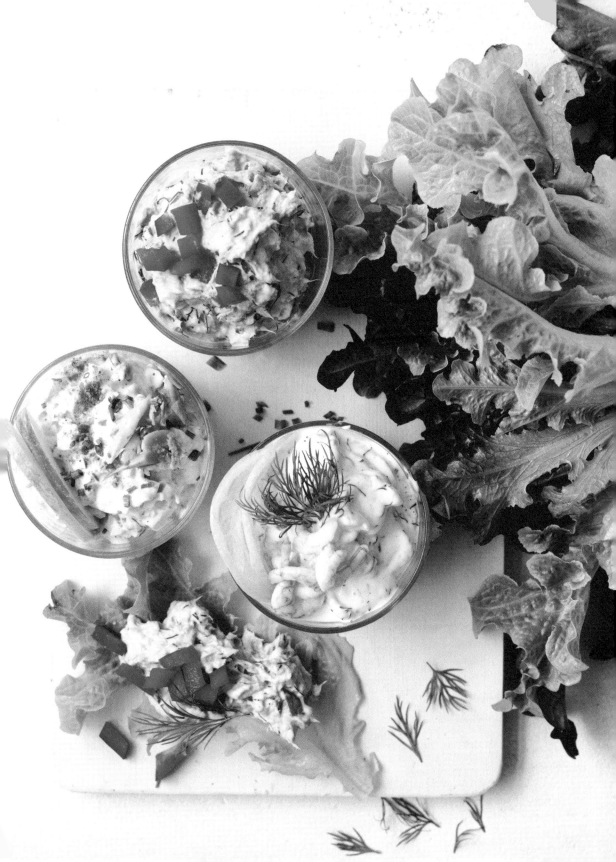

ZUCCHINI PASTA WITH PESTO

SERVES 2

1 medium-size zucchini

9 oz (250 g) cherry tomatoes in a variety of colors

5¼ oz (150 g) feta cheese, cubed

1 tbsp olive oil

Salt and black pepper

GREEN PESTO

1 bunch basil, leaves only

1 small garlic clove

1¾ oz (75 g) pine nuts

6¾ oz (200 ml) Parmesan cheese, grated

1 tsp liquid honey

Salt and black pepper

Lemon juice

⅖ cup (100 ml) olive oil

TOPPING

Fresh basil, ⅕ cup (50 ml) toasted almond flakes, large capers

Start by making the pesto: Mix all the ingredients (except the oil) in a food processor or blender. Add the oil in a thin stream while continuing to mix. Season with salt, pepper, and some more lemon juice, if needed.

"Spiralize" the zucchini into spaghetti-like strands, or cut it into tagliatelle with a potato peeler, and then place it in a bowl. Halve the tomatoes and mix them with the feta (saving some feta for garnish), olive oil, salt, and pepper.

Portion out the zucchini pasta between plates, add a dollop of pesto to each, and mix gently. Top the zucchini with some crumbled feta, fresh basil, flaked almonds, and capers.

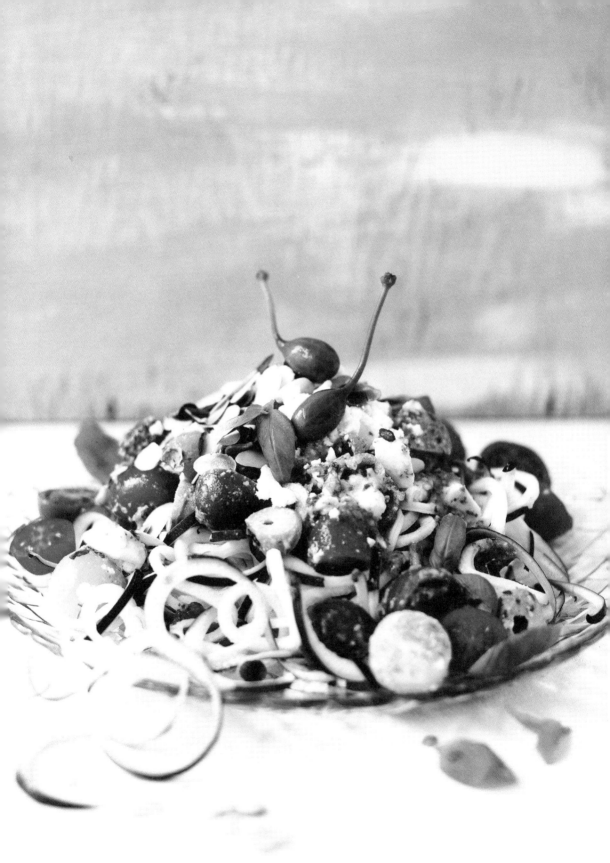

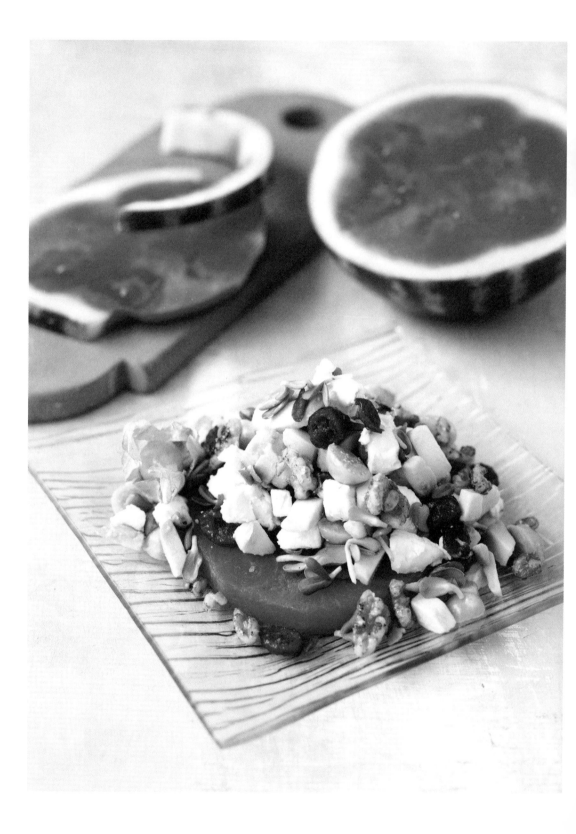

This salad makes a beautiful first course for a dinner party, or a refreshing, light lunch. Melon and chèvre cheese go very well together.

MELON SALAD WITH CHÈVRE AND AVOCADO

SERVES 1

1 slice watermelon

1 oz (28 g) sunflower sprouts

½ avocado

8 ground-cherries

1 oz (28 g) chèvre cheese, crumbled

2 tbsp dried cranberries

1 tsp olive oil

Salt and black pepper

3 walnuts, coarsely chopped

Place the slice of melon on a plate. Snip some of the green parts from the sprouts and place in a bowl. Finely dice the avocado, and halve the ground-cherries. Mix everything in the bowl. Add in the crumbled chèvre, cranberries, oil, salt, and pepper.

Mix everything together, and top the melon slice with some of the mixture. Sprinkle with walnuts.

MOZZARELLA SALAD WITH CHIOGGIA BEETS

SERVES 2

2 packets (4½ oz each) buffalo mozzarella

1 tbsp olive oil

Salt and black pepper

Grated zest of 1 lemon

9 oz (250 g) cherry tomatoes

3 Chioggia beets

1 avocado

POMEGRANATE DRESSING

Seeds from ½ pomegranate

2 tbsp olive oil

1 tbsp liquid honey

Salt and black pepper

TOPPING

1 packet sandwich cress, snipped

Seeds from ½ pomegranate

Start by making the dressing: Put the pomegranate seeds in a food processor or a blender. Add oil and honey and process until the dressing becomes smooth. Season with salt and pepper.

Place the mozzarella on a serving platter. Drizzle with the oil, season with salt and pepper, and sprinkle on the grated lemon peel. Halve the tomatoes and place them around the platter. Slice the Chioggia beets thinly with a mandolin, and cut the avocado into slices.

Place the beets and avocado around the cheese and top with snipped cress and pomegranate seeds. Serve with the dressing.

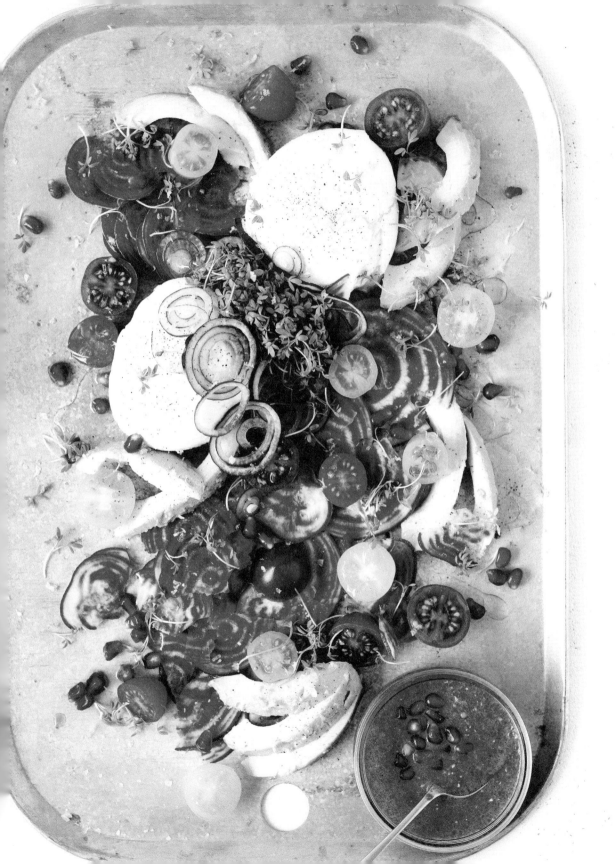

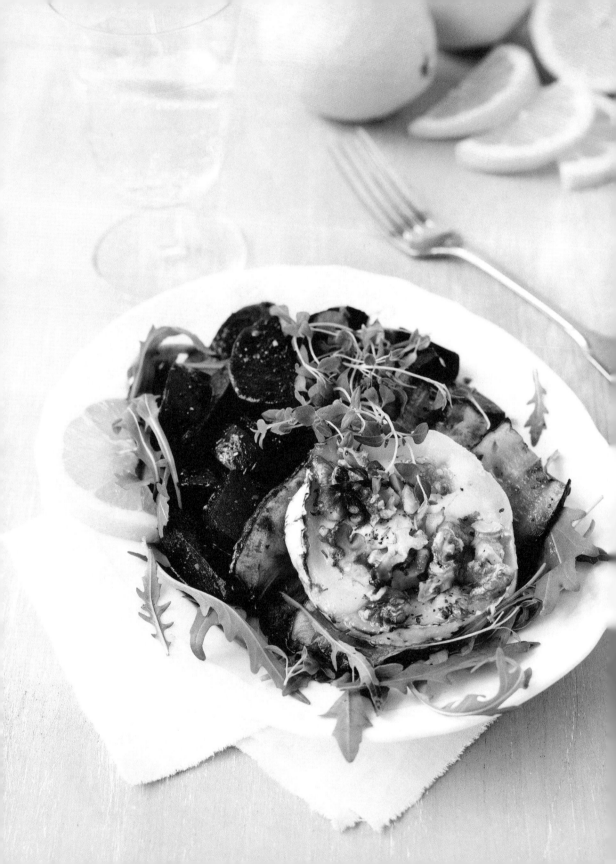

MARINATED BEETS WITH CHÈVRE GRATIN

SERVES 2

½ zucchini

1 tsp olive oil

Salt and black pepper

2 slices chèvre
   (1¾ oz each)

2 tsp liquid honey

⅛ tsp dried garden herb
   blend* (store-bought)

10 walnuts, coarsely
   chopped

1 oz (25 g) arugula

2 slices lemon

Fresh thyme

MARINATED BEETS

14 oz (400 g) beets

½ tbsp olive oil

1 tsp liquid honey

½ tbsp vinegar

⅛ tsp garden herb blend
   (store-bought)

Salt and black pepper

Start by preparing the beets: Boil them in water until soft, about 25–30 minutes. Rinse in cold water, and peel. Slice the beets and put them in a bowl. Add the remaining ingredients.

Preheat the oven to 480°F (250°C), set to bake. Slice the zucchini lengthwise, and sauté in a skillet with some oil for a minute or two. Transfer the slices to a baking sheet and season with salt and pepper. Place the chèvre on top, drizzle with honey, and sprinkle with the herbs and walnuts. Bake on the middle rack of the oven for 5 minutes.

Place arugula on two plates, and portion out the marinated beets. Place the baked zucchini and chèvre on top, and garnish with sliced lemon and fresh thyme.

*Garden herb blend (store-bought): onion, black pepper, parsley, mustard seeds, bell pepper, rosemary, Mediterranean oregano, basil, marjoram, coriander, thyme, savory

CHICKEN WRAPPED IN RICE PAPER

SERVES 4

12½ oz (350 g) boneless chicken breasts

Salt and white pepper

1 tbsp olive oil

½ tbsp fresh ginger, grated

½ small garlic clove, grated

1 tbsp soy sauce

1 fresh mango

1 avocado

1 carrot

1 salad onion

⅘ cup (200 ml) red cabbage

3½ oz (100 g) sugar snap peas

12 rice papers

1¾ oz (50 g) pea shoots

2 tbsp sesame seeds

1 bunch fresh cilantro

SESAME DRESSING

2 tbsp sesame oil

2 tbsp kecap manis*

2 tbsp light soy sauce

1 tbsp fresh ginger, finely grated

½ red chili, finely chopped

1 tbsp sesame seeds

Cut the chicken into thin slices and season with salt and pepper. Heat oil in a skillet, and sauté the chicken slices with ginger and garlic for a few minutes. Drizzle with soy sauce and continue to cook until the chicken is done. Set aside.

Peel the mango, avocado, and carrot, and cut them into thin strips. Julienne the salad onion and red cabbage, and cut the sugar snap peas in thin strips lengthwise.

Soak the rice paper in water for about 30 seconds, and then set it on a cutting board. Place chicken, mango, avocado, vegetables, and pea shoots on the paper. Roll this filling up in a wrap, and set it on a plate. Repeat with the rest of the papers. Toast the sesame seeds in a dry skillet, and sprinkle them over the wraps.

Mix all the ingredients for the dressing together in a bowl. Serve the wraps with dressing on the side for dipping, or drizzle dressing over each wrap. Garnish with cilantro.

*Kecap manis: Indonesian sweet soy sauce

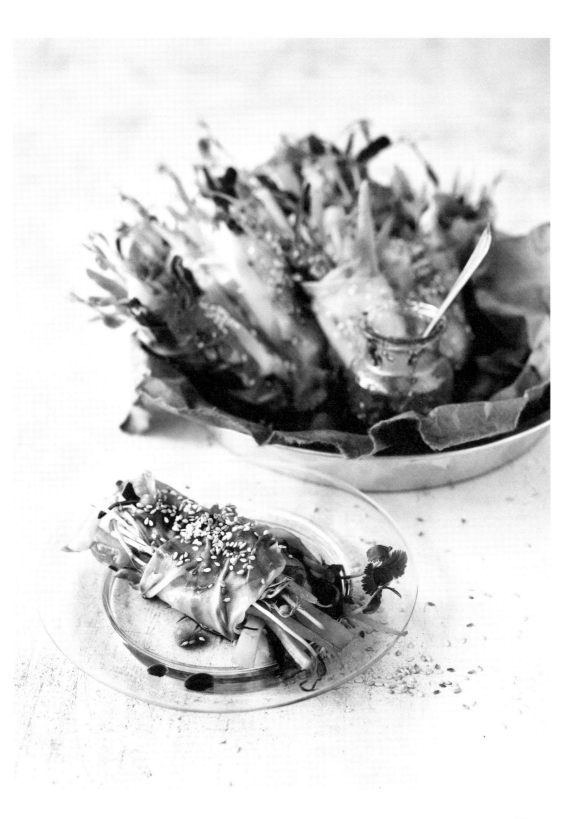

PEAR AND BLUE CHEESE SALAD

SERVES 1

½ sweet potato

1 small parsnip

1 tsp olive oil

Salt and black pepper

1 pear

1 tsp liquid honey, plus more for drizzling

1 oz (25 g) lettuce

2¾ oz (75 g) blue cheese, preferably Saint Agur

8 walnuts, coarsely chopped

1 tbsp chopped chives, for sprinkling

2 bunches red currants, or some dried cranberries, for garnish

Preheat the oven to 440°F (226°C). Cut the root vegetables into small chunks and put them on a baking sheet. Drizzle with oil, season with salt and pepper, and roast in the oven for about 15 minutes. While the root vegetables are in the oven, cut the pear into thin slices and stack the slices on top of one another. Drizzle with honey, and season with some salt and pepper. Slip the pear in the oven for the last 5 minutes of cooking.

Spread the lettuce on a plate, place the root vegetables on top, and place the pear in the middle. Cube the cheese and spread it around the vegetables.

Toast the nuts in a dry skillet, drizzle with honey, and season with salt. Toss to combine, and add it to the salad. Sprinkle the salad with chives and garnish with the red currants.

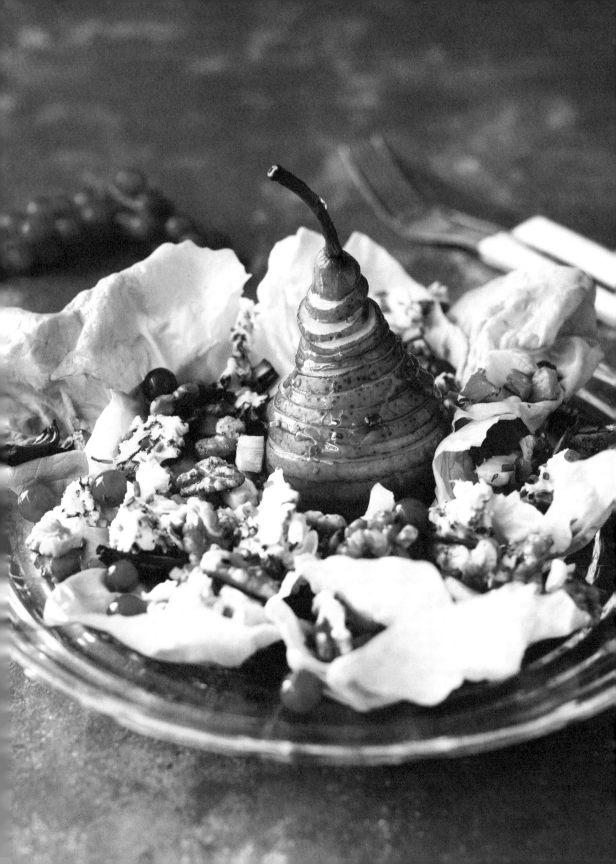

SALADS "IN A JAR"

A fun and fresh way to brown bag your lunch! Here are six variations, each one equally satisfying, tasty, and healthy. Why not make two jars at a time? You can stash them in the fridge until it's time to eat; they'll keep well for 2 to 3 days.

ASIAN SALAD

SERVES 2

⅖ cup (100 ml) spinach leaves, chopped

Some pea shoots

1 carrot, grated

½ fresh mango, sliced

2½ oz (75 g) shrimp, in brine

1¾ oz (50 g) sugar snap peas, julienned

3½ oz (100 g) seaweed noodles

2 tbsp cilantro, chopped

1 lime wedge

SESAME DRESSING

3 tbsp roasted sesame seeds

3 tbsp kecap manis

3 tbsp light soy sauce

1 tbsp rapeseed oil

1 tbsp sesame oil

1 tbsp fresh ginger, grated

½ small garlic clove, crushed

½ red chili pepper, chopped

Begin with the dressing: Mix all the ingredients in a bowl.

Layer the bottom of a glass jar with spinach. Add the pea shoots, grated carrot, sliced mango, shrimp, and julienned sugar snap peas.

Rinse the seaweed noodles and place them in a bowl; mix in one-fourth of the dressing. Transfer the noodles to the glass jar and top with the chopped cilantro. Serve with a wedge of lime.

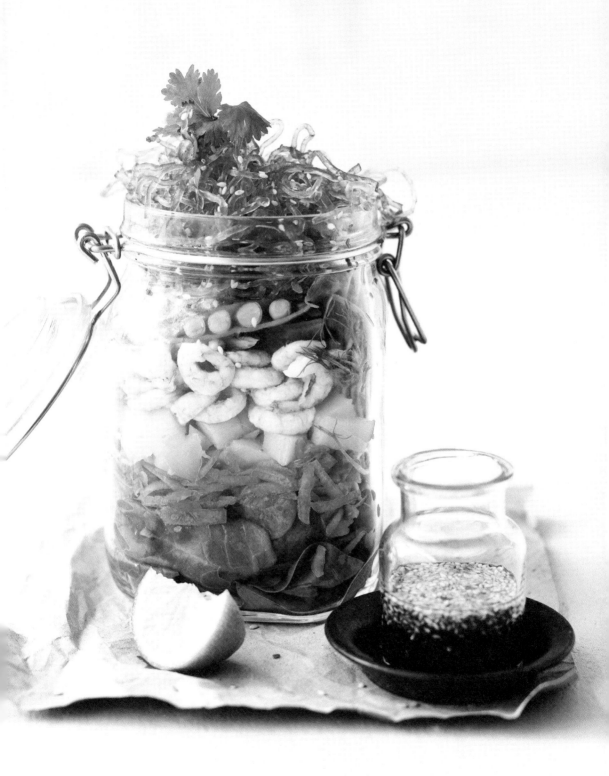

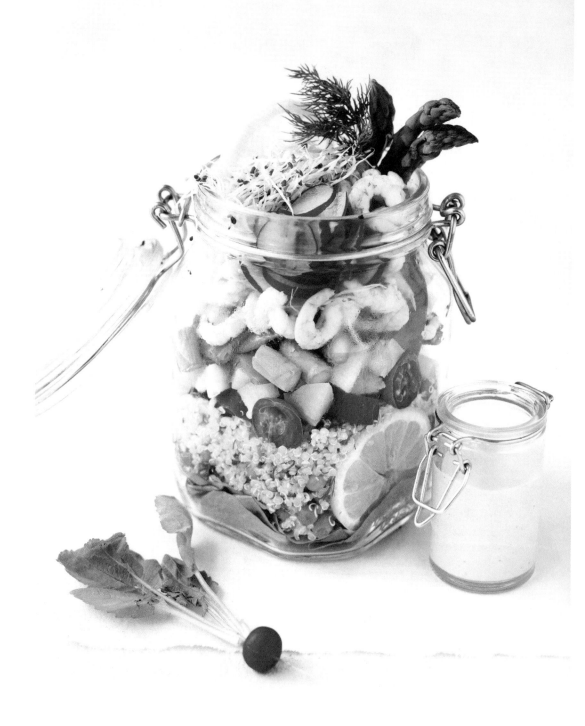

SWEDISH SALAD

SERVES 1

2¾ oz (75 g) shrimp in brine

⅖ cup (100 ml) leaf spinach, chopped

⅖ cup (100 ml) quinoa salad with lemon (see recipe on the right)

5 cherry tomatoes, halved

½ yellow bell pepper, chopped

3 lightly cooked asparagus stalks, cut into chunks

6 sugar snap peas, julienned

3 radishes, julienned

Sprouts, a small bunch of dill, and a slice of lemon, for garnish

QUINOA SALAD WITH LEMON

SERVES 1

⅖ cup (100 ml) white quinoa

Juice from ½ lemon

2 tbsp dill, chopped

⅕ cup (50 ml) frozen green peas

Salt and black pepper

TO SERVE

2 tbsp store-bought mango-chili sauce (or your favorite dressing)

Start with the quinoa salad: Cook the quinoa according to the instructions on the package. Drain the quinoa in a sieve, rinse thoroughly with water, and drain again. Transfer the quinoa to a bowl and mix in the remaining ingredients.

Pour off the brine from the shrimp. Layer the bottom of a glass jar with spinach. Add the quinoa salad and the rest of the ingredients on top of the spinach. Top it all with the sprouts, dill, and slice of lemon. Serve with mango-chili sauce.

ITALIAN SALAD

⅘ cup (200 ml) arugula

1 portion quinoa salad with sun-dried tomato (see recipe on the right)

¼ red onion, sliced

½ yellow bell pepper, chopped

5 cherry tomatoes

4½ oz (125 g) mozzarella balls

1 tbsp finely chopped red onion

1 tbsp pine nuts, toasted

Fresh basil

2 tbsp green pesto

QUINOA SALAD WITH SUN-DRIED TOMATO
SERVES 1

⅖ cup (100 ml) white quinoa

4 sun-dried tomatoes in oil, chopped

2 tbsp fresh basil, chopped

½ tsp dried garden herb blend (store-bought)

Salt and black pepper

Start with the quinoa salad: Cook the quinoa according to instructions on the package. Drain the quinoa in a sieve, rinse thoroughly with water, and drain again. Transfer the quinoa to a bowl and mix in the remaining ingredients.

Layer the bottom of a glass jar with arugula. Add the quinoa salad and the rest of the ingredients. Top everything with fresh basil and pesto.

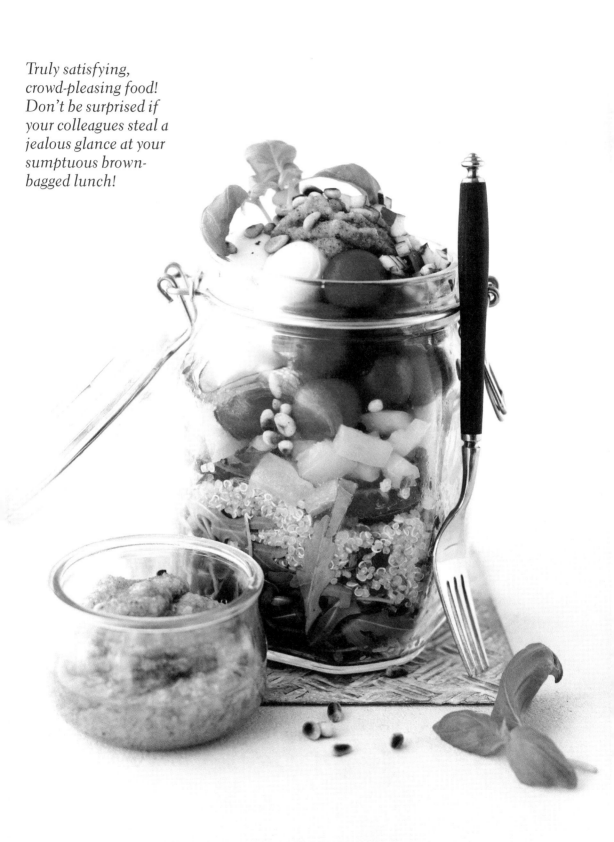

Truly satisfying, crowd-pleasing food! Don't be surprised if your colleagues steal a jealous glance at your sumptuous brown-bagged lunch!

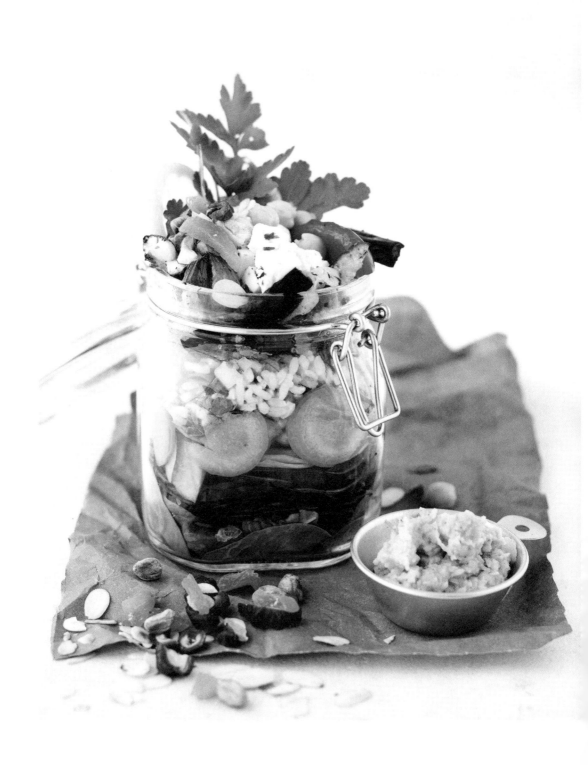

ARABIAN SALAD

SERVES 1

⅘ cup (200 ml) leaf spinach, chopped

⅘ cup (200 ml) red cabbage, julienned

1 carrot, thinly sliced

1 portion rice tabouleh (see recipe, on right)

1 portion roasted vegetables (see recipe on the right)

2¾ oz (75 g) feta cheese, diced

TOPPING

Slice of lemon, parsley, chopped pistachio nuts, toasted flaked almonds, chopped dried apricots, and dates

HUMMUS

MAKES ABOUT 4 SERVINGS

14 oz (400 g) can of chickpeas

1 small garlic clove

2 tbsp chopped Italian parsley

Juice from ½ lemon

⅕ tsp ground cumin

Salt and black pepper

⅕ cup (50 ml) olive oil

RICE TABOULEH

SERVES 2

⅖ cup (100 ml) brown rice

Juice from ½ lemon

⅕ cup (50 ml) finely chopped Italian parsley

Salt and black pepper

2 inches (5 cm) English hot house cucumber, cut into small pieces

1 tomato, cut in small pieces

½ red onion, finely chopped

ROASTED VEGETABLES

SERVES 2

½ red bell pepper, sliced

¼ eggplant, sliced

¼ zucchini, sliced

½ red onion, in segments

½ tbsp olive oil

Salt and black pepper

½ tsp dried garden herb blend (store-bought)

Start by making the hummus: Mix all the ingredients (saving a few chickpeas for the garnish) in a food processor, and season with salt and pepper. Refrigerate.

Cook the rice for the tabouleh according to the instructions on the package. Stir in the remaining ingredients. Set aside.

Preheat the oven to 440°F (226°C). Transfer the vegetables and the onion to a rimmed baking sheet. Drizzle with oil and season with salt, pepper, and dried herbs blend. Mix and roast in the oven for about 15 minutes.

Line the bottom of a glass jar with spinach. Add red cabbage and carrot, rice tabouleh, and roasted vegetables on top. Top it off with feta cheese, chickpeas, slice of lemon, parsley, pistachios, flaked almonds, apricots, and dates. Serve with the hummus.

This is raw food at its best! It's full of wonderful flavor, and loaded with digestive enzymes that will help your hormonal balance.

RAW FOOD SALAD

SERVES 1

⅖ cup (100 ml) spinach leaves, chopped

1 portion cauliflower rice (see recipe below)

Pomegranate seeds

½ mango, cut into chunks

1 portion lemon-infused broccoli (see recipe on the right)

⅖ cup (100 ml) red cabbage, julienned

⅖ cup (100 ml) watermelon, diced

½ avocado, cut into chunks

Some sprouts, for garnish

CAULIFLOWER RICE
SERVES 2

½ head cauliflower

Juice from ½ lemon

2 tbsp chopped parsley

Salt and black pepper

LEMON-INFUSED BROCCOLI
SERVES 2

½ bunch broccoli, florets only

1 tbsp olive oil

Juice from ½ lemon

LEMON DRESSING
SERVES 2

Juice from ½ lemon

1 tsp liquid honey

1 tbsp olive oil

Salad seasoning

Start by making the cauliflower rice: Grate the cauliflower coarsely on a box grater, and place it in a bowl. Mix it with lemon juice, parsley, salt, and pepper.

Cut the broccoli florets into small pieces, and place them in another bowl. Drizzle with oil and lemon juice, and mix.

Mix all the ingredients for the dressing in a bowl.

Cover the bottom of a glass jar with spinach leaves. Layer the cauliflower rice, pomegranate seeds, mango, broccoli, red cabbage, and melon, ending with avocado. Top with sprouts, and drizzle with lemon dressing.

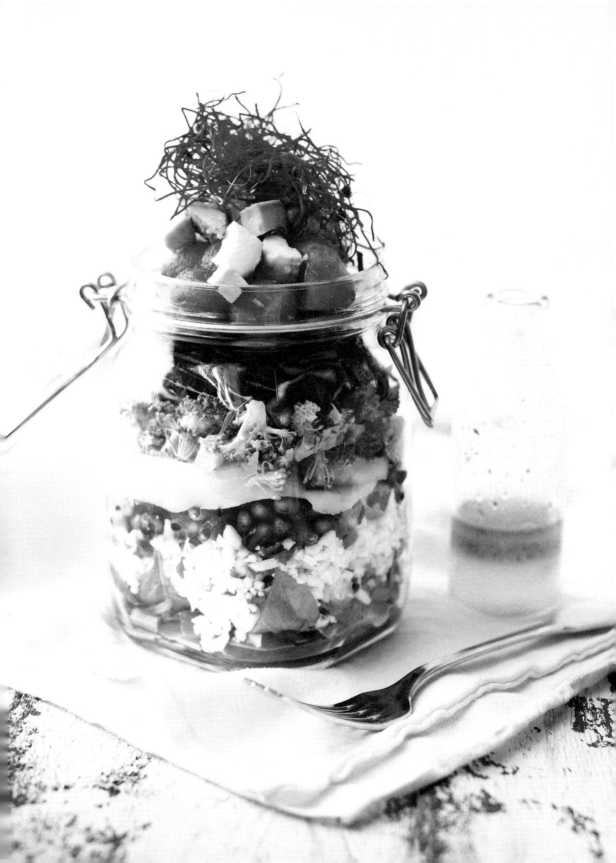

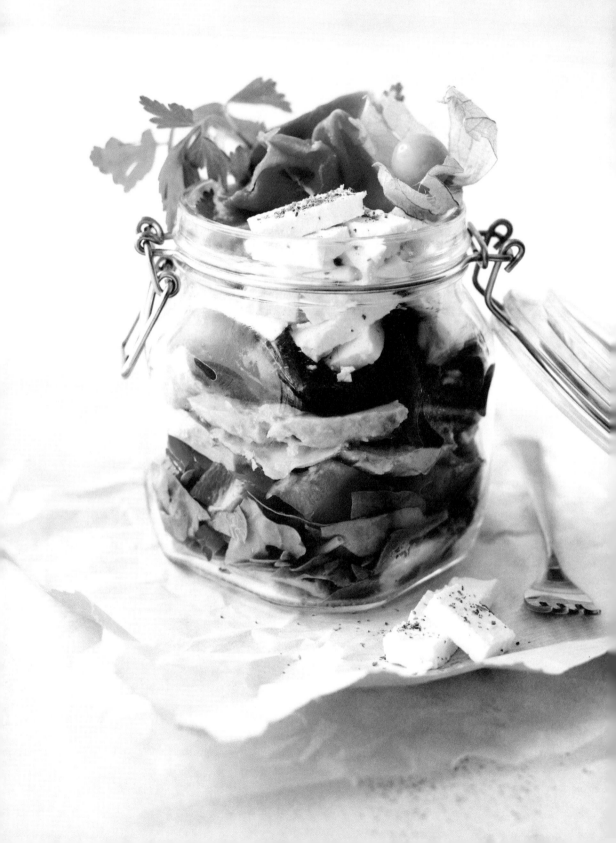

MEDITERRANEAN SALAD

SERVES 1

⅖ cup (100 ml) spinach
leaves, chopped

⅖ cup (100 ml) red bell
pepper

½ avocado, sliced

1 portion marinated beets
(see recipe below)

2¾ oz (75 g) feta cheese

2 slices Serrano ham

MARINATED BEETS

SERVES 2

14 oz (400 g) beets

½ tbsp olive oil

1 tsp liquid honey

1 tbsp balsamic vinegar

⅛ tsp dried garden herb
blend (store-bought)

Salt and black pepper

VINAIGRETTE DRESSING

SERVES 2

2 tbsp olive oil

1 tsp liquid honey

1 tbsp balsamic vinegar

⅛ tsp Italian salad
seasoning

1 tbsp water

TOPPING

Ground-cherries and
parsley

Start by preparing the beets: Boil them in water until soft, about 25–30 minutes. Rinse under cold water, peel, slice, and place them in a bowl. Mix in the remaining ingredients.

Cover the bottom of a glass jar with chopped spinach. Layer bell pepper, avocado, marinated beets, and feta cheese. Top with Serrano ham, and garnish with ground cherries and parsley.

Mix all the ingredients for the dressing in a bowl, and drizzle some dressing over the salad.

OMELET WRAP WITH A SELECTION OF FILLINGS

A plain omelet with salad and your favorite dip. It's an easy lunch that's perfect for bringing along on a trip, or to work!

BASIC OMELET RECIPE
SERVES 1

2 eggs

Salt and pepper

1 tsp butter or oil

Whisk together the eggs, salt, and pepper in a bowl. Pour the mixture into a medium-hot skillet with butter or oil, and cook until the eggs have "settled." Transfer the omelet to a plate to cool.

   Place lettuce, maybe some type of green shoots, and some other favorite vegetables on top of the cooked omelet. Add on with one of the dips below, roll up the omelet, and pack it up for lunch.

TUNA FILLING
SERVES 2

Approx. 6½ oz (180 g) tuna in water or oil

2 tbsp mayonnaise

2 tbsp sour cream*

1 tbsp hot and sweet mustard

⅕ cup (50 ml) leek, julienned

½ bell pepper, diced

2 tbsp chopped parsley

Salt and black pepper

Mix all the ingredients in a bowl. Season with salt and pepper.

SHRIMP FILLING
SERVES 2

⅘ cup (200 ml) shrimp

2 tbsp mayonnaise

2 tbsp cultured cream*

1 tbsp chopped dill

¼ red onion, finely chopped

Salt and black pepper

Some freshly squeezed lemon juice

Mix all the ingredients in a bowl. Season with salt, pepper, and some freshly squeezed lemon juice.

CHICKEN FILLING
SERVES 2

9 oz (250 g) grilled chicken

2 tbsp mayonnaise

2 tbsp sour cream*

1 tsp curry powder

⅕ tsp turmeric

⅕ cup (50 ml) leek, julienned

½ diced apple

2 tbsp chopped parsley

Salt and black pepper

Slice the chicken into thin strips, and mix with the rest of the ingredients in a bowl. Season with salt and pepper.

*Swedish cultured cream; full-fat sour cream works here

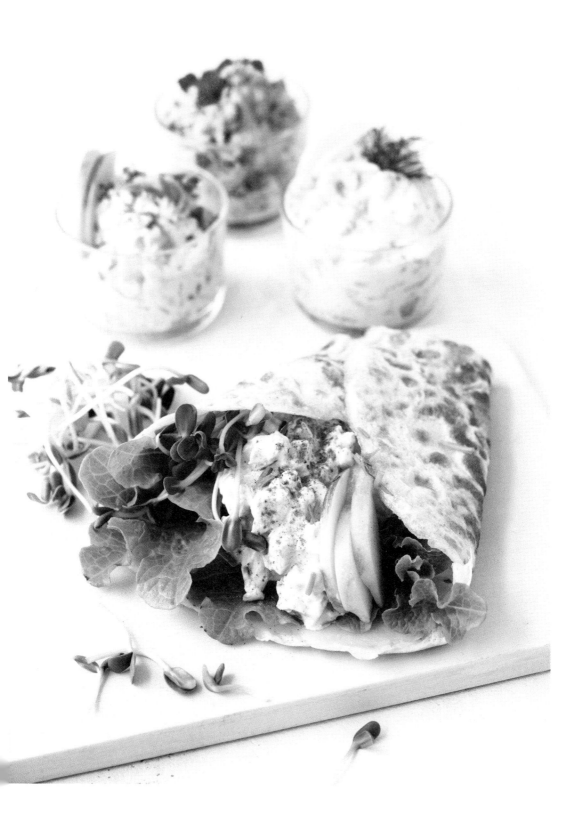

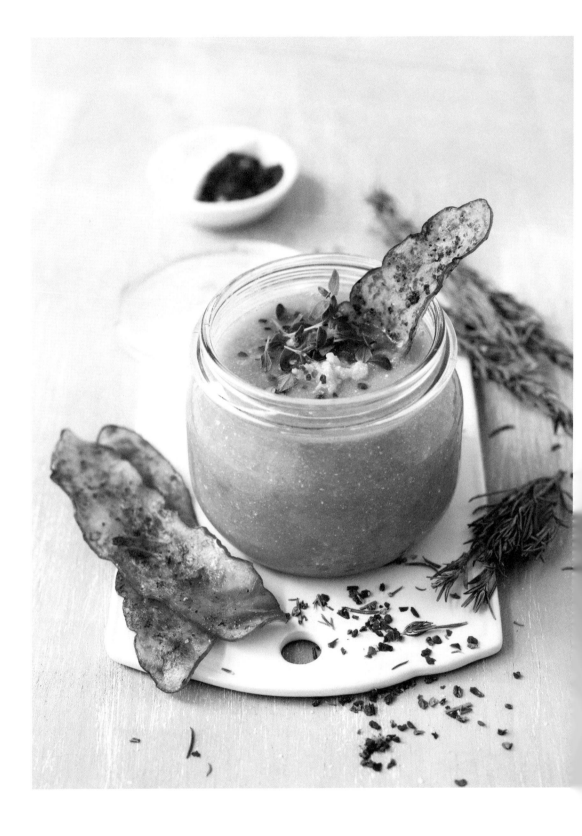

CARROT SOUP WITH GINGER AND CHICKEN BACON

SERVES 4

1⅓ lb (500 g) carrots

1 yellow onion

2 garlic cloves

1 tbsp olive oil

3½ cups (800 ml) water

2 tbsp grated fresh ginger

1 tbsp liquid honey

1 tbsp organic stock powder

1 tsp dried garden herb blend (store-bought)

⅓ tsp turmeric

A pinch of chili flakes

Salt and black pepper

TOPPING

Dried or fresh herbs— rosemary or oregano, for example

8 slices fried chicken bacon

Peel and thinly slice the carrots. Chop the onion and garlic. Heat some oil in a large saucepan and sauté the onion and garlic for a few minutes. Add the remaining ingredients and bring to a boil. Cook for about 10 minutes.

Blend the soup till smooth in a food processor or a blender, and pour it back into the saucepan. Bring it back to a simmer and dilute it with more water, if needed. Season with salt and pepper. Ladle the soup into bowls and top with fresh herbs and slices of chicken bacon.

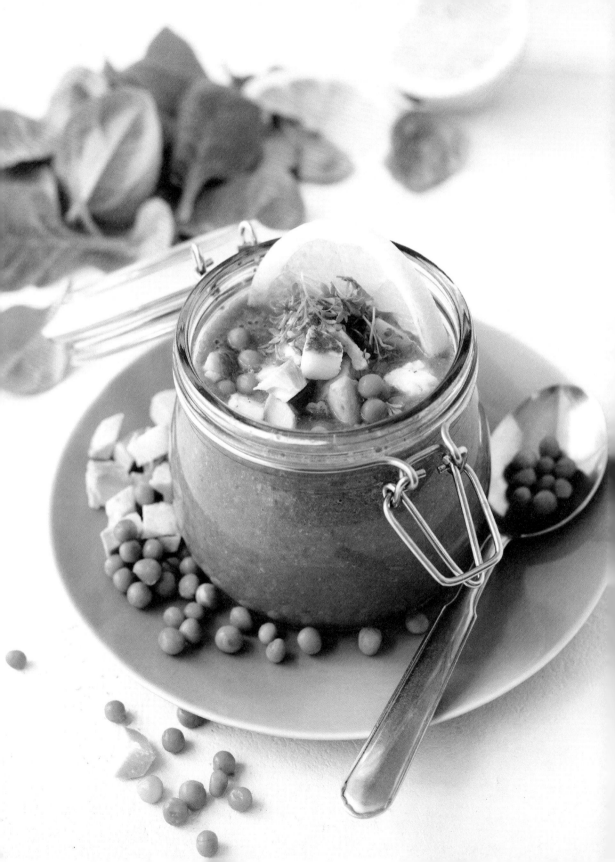

SPINACH SOUP WITH AVOCADO AND GREEN PEAS

SERVES 2

½ small onion

1 small garlic clove

½ tbsp olive oil

5¼ oz (150 g) fresh
 spinach

2⅓ cups (500 ml) water

1 cube organic vegetable
 stock

Salt and pepper

⅖ cup (100 ml) green
 peas

½ avocado

Juice from ½ lemon

TOPPING

1 oz (30 g) fried halloumi
 cheese, ⅕ cup (50 ml)
 green peas, sandwich
 cress and lemon slices

Chop onion and garlic. Heat some oil in a large saucepan and cook the onion and garlic for a few minutes. Add the spinach, water, stock cube, salt, and pepper. Let it boil for about 5 minutes. Add peas, avocado, and lemon juice.

Blend the soup till smooth in a food processor or a blender, and season with salt and pepper. Ladle the soup into bowls, and top the soup with halloumi cheese, peas, cress, and lemon.

TOMATO SOUP WITH HALLOUMI CHEESE

SERVES 2

½ small onion

1 small garlic clove

1 tsp olive oil

7 oz (200 g) crushed
    tomatoes

1 tsp dried garden herb
    blend (store-bought)

1 cube organic vegetable
    stock

1 tsp liquid honey

1¼ cups (300 ml) water

Salt and black pepper

TOPPING

3½ oz (100 g) halloumi
    cheese

1 tsp olive oil

Fresh oregano

Chop the onion and garlic. Heat the oil in a large saucepan and cook the onion for a few minutes. Add the crushed tomatoes, dried herb blend, stock cube, honey, and water. Bring to a boil, and season with salt and pepper.

Blend the soup till smooth in a food processor or blender, and pour it back into the saucepan. Let it cook another 5 minutes. Dilute it with more water, if needed.

Cut the halloumi into chunks. Heat the oil in a skillet and fry the cheese for a few minutes. Ladle the soup into bowls, and top it with the halloumi and fresh oregano.

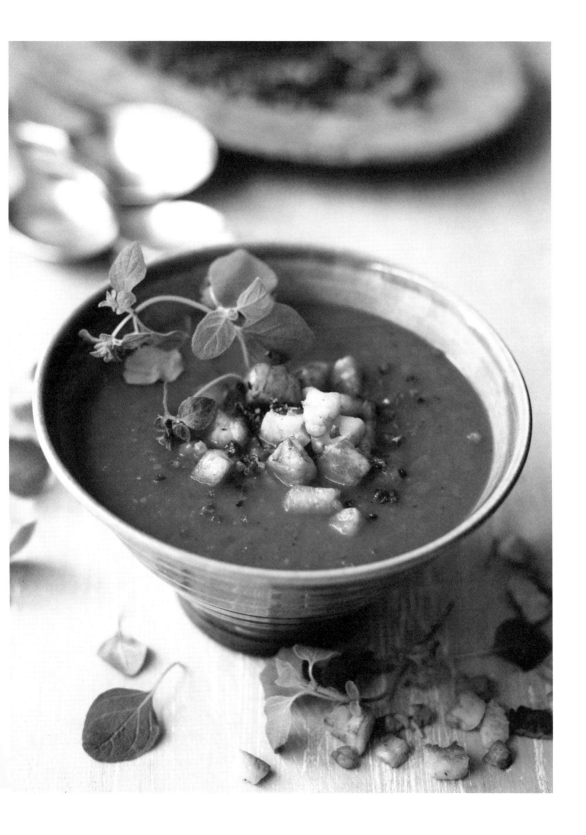

ASIAN SALMON SOUP WITH SEAGRASS NOODLES

SERVES 2

1 garlic clove

2 salad onions

½ tbsp olive oil

1 tbsp grated fresh ginger

2½ cups (600 ml) water

1 cube organic fish stock

1 tbsp kecap manis

1 tsp fish sauce

1 tbsp light soy sauce

1 carrot

10 cremini mushrooms

4½ oz (125 g) bok choy

7 oz (200 g) salmon filet

¼ bunch broccoli, florets only

3½ oz (100 g) seagrass noodles

½ bunch cilantro

TOPPING

2 tbsp dried cranberries

2 tbsp peanuts

Fresh coriander

Wedges of lime

Finely chop the garlic and salad onions. Heat the oil in a large saucepan and sauté the garlic, salad onions, and ginger for a minute or two. Add water and stock cube. Stir in the kecap manis, fish sauce, and soy sauce. Bring to a boil and let simmer for 10 minutes.

Thinly slice the carrot. Slice the mushrooms, bok choy, and salmon. Carefully add it all to the saucepan, along with the broccoli, and let everything simmer for another few minutes.

Rinse the noodles and add them to the soup. Season with salt and pepper. Chop the cilantro and add it to the soup.

Ladle the soup into bowls and top with cranberries, peanuts, coriander, and wedges of lime.

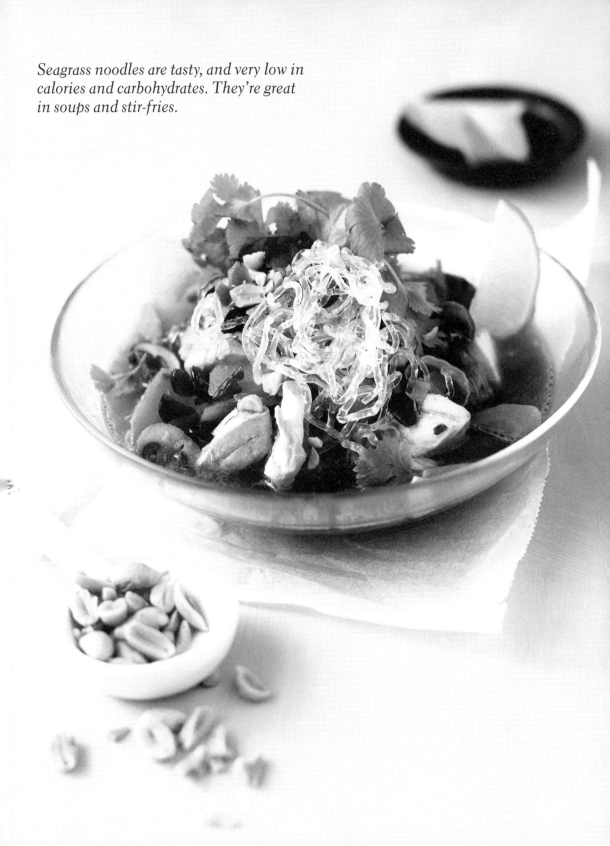

Seagrass noodles are tasty, and very low in calories and carbohydrates. They're great in soups and stir-fries.

FERMENTED VEGETABLES WITH TURMERIC

MAKES 1 JAR

1 carrot

1 parsnip

1 red onion

5 radishes

½ bunch broccoli

½ head cauliflower

1 tbsp iodine-free salt

1 tsp yellow mustard seeds

1 tsp dark mustard seeds

1 tbsp turmeric

Rinse all the vegetables thoroughly, and cut them into pieces. Place everything in a bowl. Mix in the salt. Let stand for 2 hours.

Mix in the mustard seeds and turmeric. Place the mixture in a glass jar and press down on the contents so they're well packed. Leave ¾ inch of air space at the top. Screw on a tight-fitting lid and put the jar on a tray.

Store the jar in a dark place, preferably the pantry at room temperature. Open the jar once a day and check the fermentation. It will begin to bubble in the jar after 1–2 days. Once it stops hissing when you open the lid, the process is starting to settle, at which point you won't need to open the jar anymore. Add salt water (1 tbsp salt per quart of water) if the level of liquid falls.

Your fermented vegetables will be ready after a few days. They can stay at room temperature for a week, but must be stored in the refrigerator afterward, where they will keep for several months.

SAUERKRAUT WITH APPLE AND CARA-WAY SEED

MAKES 1 LARGE JAR

1 white cabbage, approx. 2¼ lb (1 kg)

1 tbsp iodine-free salt

1 red apple

1 tbsp whole caraway seeds

Julienne the white cabbage very finely and place it in a bowl. Mix in the salt. Let it sit for several hours.

Rinse the apple thoroughly, grate it coarsely, and mix it into the white cabbage along with the caraway seeds. Transfer everything to a glass jar and press down the contents until they're well packed. Leave ¾ inch of air space at the top. Screw on a tight-fitting lid and set the jar on a tray.

Store the jar in a dark area like the pantry. Open the jar once a day to check the fermentation. After 2–3 days it will begin to bubble in the jar. When it no longer hisses when you open the jar, the process has settled and you no longer need to open the jar every day. Add salt water (1 tbsp salt per quart of water) if the level of liquid drops.

The sauerkraut will be ready after a few days. It can stay at room temperature for about a week, and then it must be stored in the refrigerator, where it will keep for several months.

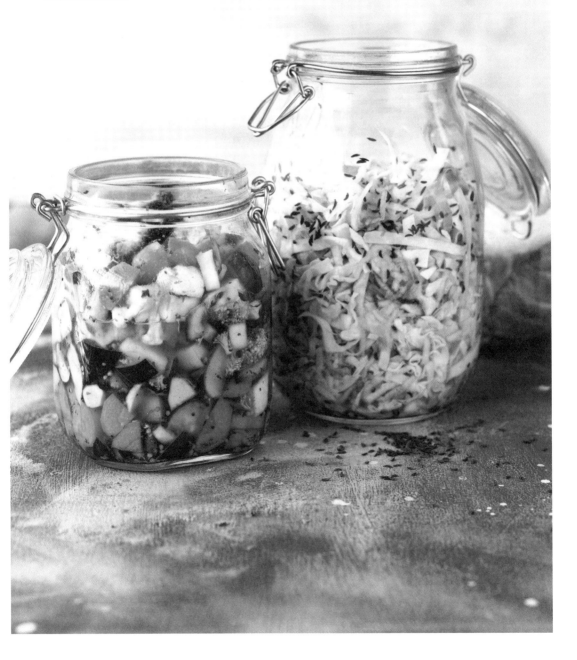

Be extremely careful with cleanliness when you ferment foods yourself. Tools, hands, and jars need to be immaculate.

MAIN DISHES

*Easy to prepare, tasty, healthful, and full of energy—
that's what characterizes the main dishes in this chapter.
Enjoy meals that include fish, shellfish, poultry, meat,
and vegetables; they're all highly satisfying and contribute
to a fine balance in the body, while having little impact
on blood glucose levels.*

Fruity rice stir-fry with seared salmon and aioli 116 * Pike-perch with lemon-sautéed
vegetables and pea pesto 118 * Chèvre-stuffed salmon with pesto and ajvar quinoa 121
* Meatloaf with oven-roasted tomatoes 122 * Italian chicken pot 124 * Sirloin steak with
romesco sauce and lentil salad 127 * Cod roulades with mango salsa 128 * Fish soup 131
* Ulrika's Persian lamb stew 132 * Cauliflower rice with curried chicken 135 * Gluten-free
tortilla wraps with chicken and papaya 136 * Portabella mushroom with ajvar relish and
turkey breast 139 * Meatballs with cauliflower risotto 140

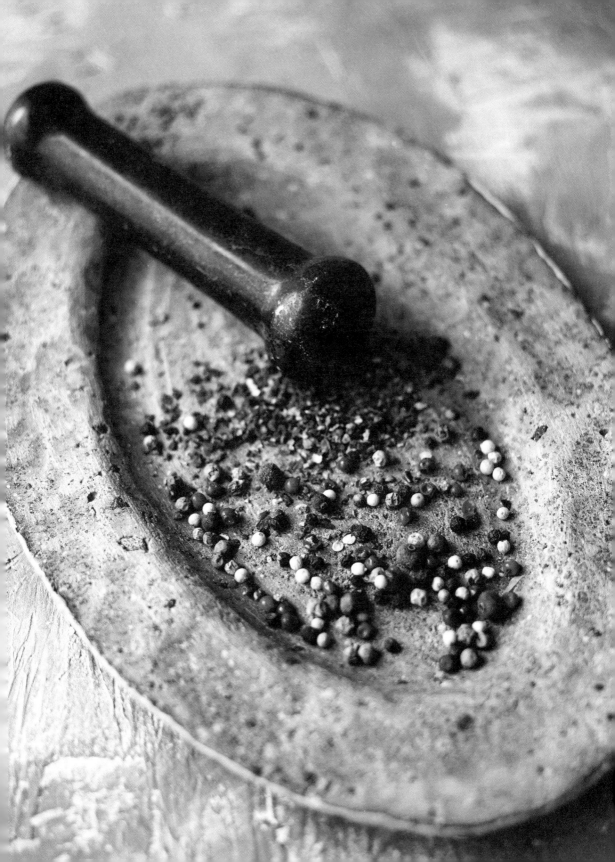

FRUITY RICE STIR-FRY WITH SEARED SALMON AND AIOLI

SERVES 2

⅖ cup (100 ml) cooked brown rice

1 salad onion

1 carrot

½ red bell pepper

3½ oz (100 g) sugar snap peas

1 tbsp olive oil, divided

⅖ cup (100 ml) chopped red cabbage

1 tbsp freshly grated ginger

½ small garlic clove, grated

Salt and black pepper

Freshly squeezed lemon juice, to taste

10½ oz (300 g) salmon filet

½ mango

1 tsp sesame seeds

Fresh cilantro

1 passion fruit

TO SERVE

Bok choy leaves that have been quickly dipped in boiling water

Seagrass salad and aioli (store-bought from the deli)

Boil the rice according to the instructions on the packaging. Cut the salad onion into thin slices. Cut the carrot and bell pepper into small chunks. Julienne the sugar snap peas.

Heat ½ tbsp oil in a skillet and stir-fry the rice, salad onion, carrot, bell pepper, sugar snap peas, red cabbage, ginger, and garlic for a few minutes. Season with salt, pepper, and some lemon juice. Keep warm.

Slice the salmon and sprinkle with salt and pepper. Heat ½ tbsp oil in a skillet or grill pan, and sear the fish for a few minutes on each side until it's cooked through.

Place the stir-fried rice on plates and place a piece of salmon on top. Slice part of the mango, and dice the rest finely. Place the diced mango on the stir-fried rice. Scatter with sesame seeds and top with fresh cilantro. Garnish with slices of mango and passion fruit, and serve it with bok choy, seagrass salad, and aioli.

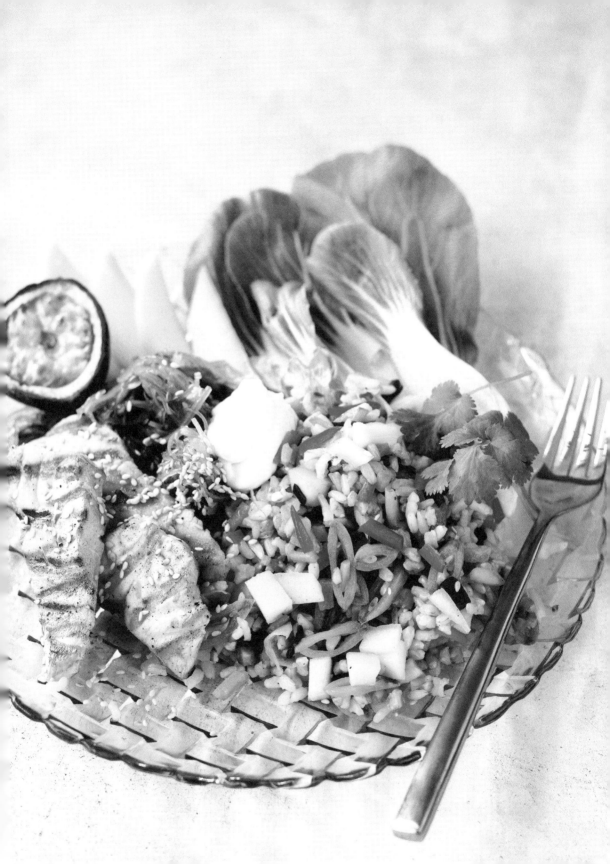

PIKE-PERCH WITH LEMON-SAUTÉED VEGETABLES AND PEA PESTO

SERVES 2

10½–14 oz (300–400 g) filet of pike-perch

Salt and white pepper

2 tbsp butter, divided

1 large carrot

7 oz (200 g) soy beans

Salt and black pepper

Zest and juice from ½ lemon

2 tbsp chopped fresh dill

1 bunch green asparagus

PEA PESTO

3½ oz (100 g) blanched almonds

⅘ cup (200 ml) frozen peas

Juice from 1 lemon

1 garlic clove

⅖ cup (100 ml) olive or rapeseed oil

Salt and black pepper

TOPPING

Chili flakes

Toasted, flaked almonds

Lemon wedges

Sprigs of fresh dill

Preheat the oven to 350°F (175°C). Start on the pea pesto: Place almonds, peas, lemon juice, and garlic in a food processor or blender. Add oil a little bit at a time, and mix to make a smooth sauce. Season with salt and black pepper. Store the pesto in the refrigerator until it's time to serve.

Season the fish filets with salt and white pepper; heat up 1 tbsp butter in a skillet, and sear the filets in the hot butter for 1–2 minutes on each side. Place the filets in an ovenproof dish and cook them in the oven for about 15 minutes.

Cut the carrot into small chunks. Heat 1 tbsp butter in a skillet and sauté carrot and soy beans for a few minutes. Season with salt, black pepper, and lemon juice. Stir in the dill, and set aside.

Cook the asparagus for about 3 minutes in lightly salted water. Place the fish on a plate with the warm vegetables. Top with chili flakes, flaked almonds, lemon zest, lemon wedges, and dill. Serve along with the pea pesto.

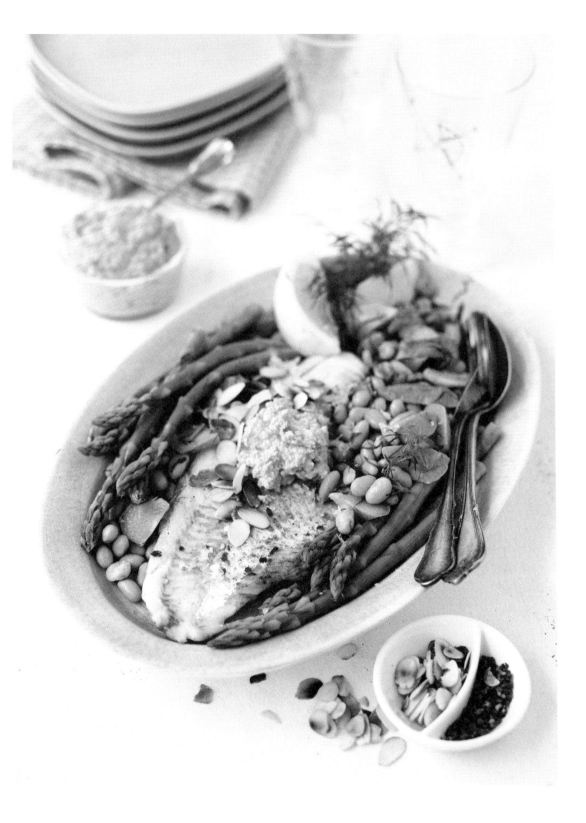

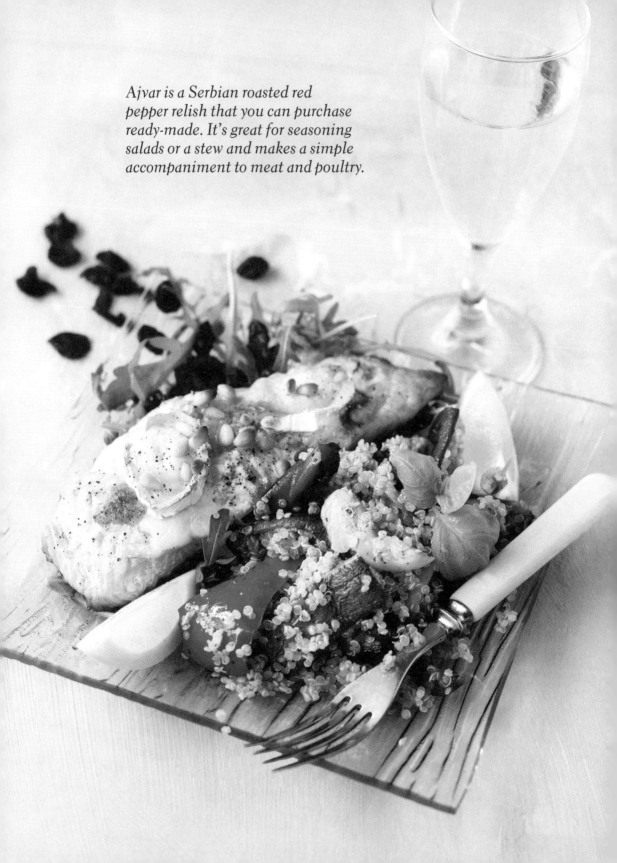

Ajvar is a Serbian roasted red pepper relish that you can purchase ready-made. It's great for seasoning salads or a stew and makes a simple accompaniment to meat and poultry.

CHÈVRE-STUFFED SALMON WITH PESTO AND AJVAR QUINOA

SERVES 4

4 salmon filets, approx.
  5¼ oz (150 g) each

4 tbsp green pesto (see
  p. 78)

3½ oz (100 g) chèvre

Salt and black pepper

1¾ oz (50 g) pine nuts

1¾ oz (50 g) arugula

AJVAR QUINOA
SERVES 4

⅘ cup (200 ml) white
  quinoa

Salt and black pepper

½ tsp dried garden herb
  blend (store-bought)

⅕ cup (50 ml) ajvar relish

½ yellow bell pepper

½ red bell pepper

1 yellow onion

¼ zucchini

1 tbsp olive oil

TOPPING

4 tbsp dried cranberries

1 lemon, cut into wedges

Fresh basil leaves

Preheat the oven to 400°F (200°C). Set the salmon filets in a dish. Make an incision into each filet and fill it with pesto and chèvre. Season with salt and freshly ground pepper, and sprinkle with pine nuts. Bake in the oven for 20 minutes, or until the salmon is cooked through.

Cook the quinoa according to the directions on the package. Drain it through a sieve; rinse thoroughly with water and drain again. Transfer the quinoa to a bowl and mix in salt, pepper, herb blend, and ajvar relish.

Cut the bell peppers in large chunks, and the onion and zucchini into slices. Heat the oil in a skillet, and sauté the vegetables for a few minutes. Season with salt and pepper. Mix the sautéed vegetables with the quinoa.

Transfer the salmon to a serving platter along with the quinoa and arugula. Garnish with dried cranberries, lemon wedges, and fresh basil.

MEATLOAF WITH OVEN-ROASTED TOMATOES

SERVES 4

1¼ lb (500 g) ground beef

1 egg

1 yellow onion

4 sun-dried tomatoes, in oil

⅖ cup (100 ml) Italian parsley, chopped

½ tsp dried garden herb blend (store-bought)

Salt and black pepper

5¼ oz (150 g) Boursin cheese, with garlic and herbs

2 tbsp pine nuts

OVEN-ROASTED TOMATOES

1¼ lb (500 g) cherry tomatoes

12 red small frying onions, or 1 large red onion

1 tbsp olive oil

⅛ tsp dried garden herb blend (store-bought)

Salt and black pepper

FOR SERVING

Arugula

Chopped Italian parsley

Preheat the oven to 400°F (200°C). Put the ground meat and egg in a bowl. Finely chop the onion, and sun-dried tomatoes. Mix everything into the ground meat along with the parsley, dried herb blend, salt, and pepper. Mix thoroughly.

Shape the meat into a loaf on a baking sheet or in a loaf pan. Press the Boursin down in the middle, and scatter the pine nuts over the loaf.

Cut half of the tomatoes in two, and place them around the loaf along with the whole tomatoes. Peel the red onions and place them among the tomatoes (if using one large onion, chop into chunks first). Drizzle olive oil over the tomatoes and onions, and season with herb blend, salt, and pepper.

Bake for about 30 minutes or until the meatloaf is cooked all the way through. Serve with arugula salad and parsley.

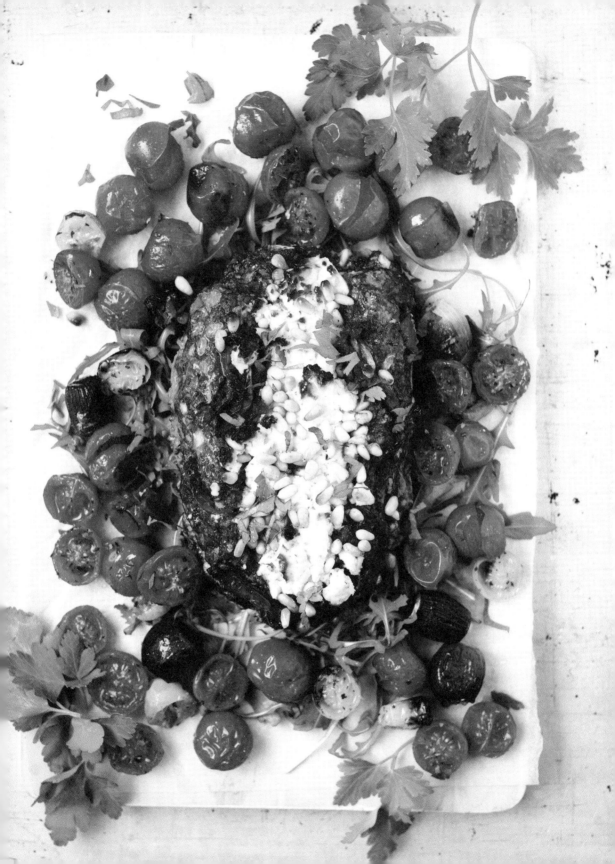

ITALIAN CHICKEN POT

SERVES 2

½ yellow onion

1 garlic clove

½ zucchini

½ red bell pepper

½ yellow bell pepper

½ fennel bulb (hard inner core removed)

6 mushrooms

2 boneless chicken breasts, approx. 5¼ oz (150 g) each

1 tsp olive oil

Dried garden herb blend (store-bought)

Salt and black pepper

2 tbsp pesto

1 tbsp organic chicken stock or 1 organic vegetable stock cube

⅖ cup (100 ml) water

⅖ cup (100 ml) oat cream (dairy-free)

6 green olives

1 tbsp chopped basil + whole leaves for garnish

Chop the onion, and mince the garlic. Cut the vegetables and mushrooms into chunks. Cut the chicken breasts into smaller pieces.

Heat the oil in a skillet and sauté everything for a few minutes. Season with herb garden blend, salt, and pepper.

Pour everything into a large pot or Dutch oven, and add in pesto, chicken stock, water, and oat cream. Let simmer over low heat for about 20 minutes. Add olives and basil. Garnish with fresh basil leaves and serve.

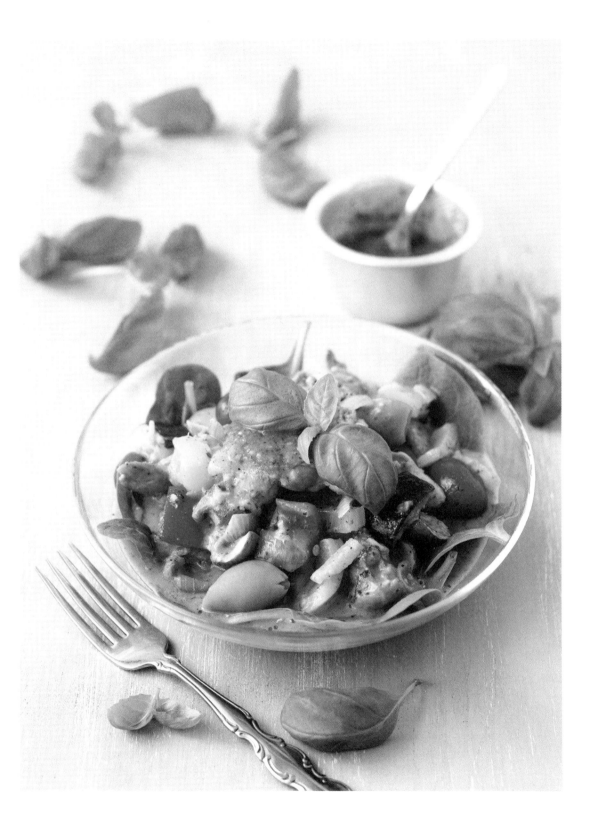

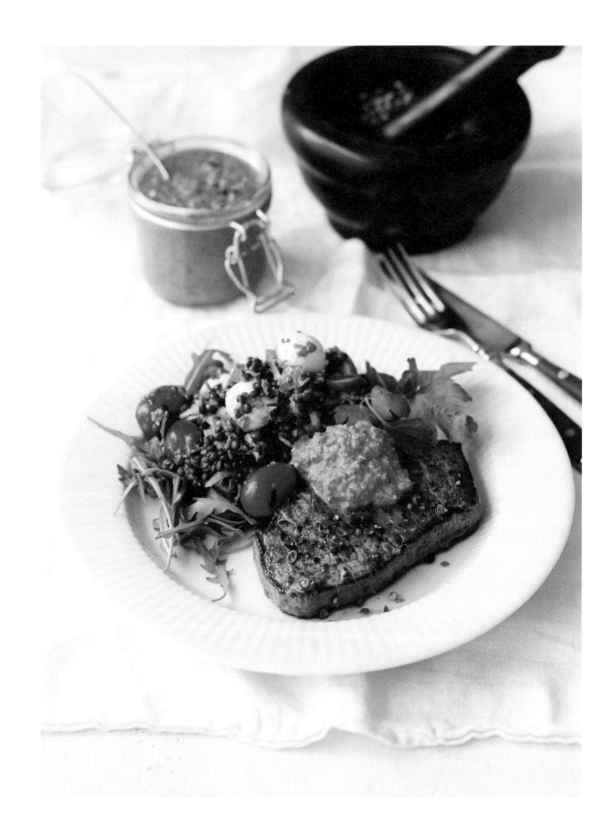

SIRLOIN STEAK WITH ROMESCO SAUCE AND LENTIL SALAD

Romesco sauce pairs well with just about everything. Any leftovers in the bowl will keep for a week in the refrigerator.

SERVES 2

⅖ cup (100 ml) Le Puy or Beluga lentils

10 cherry tomatoes

½ red onion

Salt and black pepper

1 tbsp chopped fresh parsley or basil

1 tbsp olive oil

4½ oz (125 g) mini mozzarella balls

2 slices of sirloin, about 5¼ oz (150 g) each

1 tbsp butter

1 oz (25 g) arugula

A few sprigs of parsley, for garnish

ROMESCO SALSA

3½ oz (100 g) blanched almonds

9 oz (250 g) roasted bell peppers (from a jar)

1 tbsp red wine vinegar

2 garlic cloves

1 tsp chili flakes

1 tsp salt

⅘ cup (200 ml) olive oil

⅖ cup (100 ml) rapeseed oil

Start by making the romesco sauce: Place all the ingredients (except the oils) in a food processor or blender. Puree everything to a somewhat fine chop, and add the oils in a thin stream while still blending. Store the sauce in the refrigerator until it's time to serve.

Cook the lentils according to the instructions on the packaging. Drain off the water and place the lentils in a bowl. Slice the tomatoes and finely chop the onion. Mix everything together with salt, pepper, fresh herbs, oil, and mozzarella.

Season the meat with salt and pepper. Heat the butter in a skillet and sauté the steaks on both sides for a few minutes, as desired.

Place the steaks on plates together with the lentil salad, Romesco sauce, and arugula. Garnish with a sprig of parsley, and serve.

COD ROULADES WITH MANGO SALSA

SERVES 2

10½ oz (300 g) thin cod filets

Salt and white pepper

1 tsp butter

⅖ cup (100 ml) water

7 oz (200 g) Brussels sprouts

½ tbsp olive oil

Lime wedges, for garnish

Sprigs of cilantro, for garnish

MANGO SALSA

3½ oz (100 g) shrimp, peeled

½ mango

¼ red onion

Juice from ½ lime

½ tbsp olive oil

½ red chili, finely chopped

Salt and black pepper

½ bunch fresh cilantro, chopped

Start by making the mango salsa: Put the shrimp in a bowl. Dice the mango into small pieces. Chop the red onion. Mix everything together in the bowl with lime juice and olive oil. Season with the chopped chili, salt, and pepper. Mix in the cilantro.

Season the fish with salt and pepper. Roll up the filets into roulades and secure them with toothpicks. Heat the butter in a skillet and sauté the roulades on all sides. Pour the water into the pan and let the fish simmer until it is cooked through, about 10 minutes.

Cut the Brussels sprouts in half, and stir-fry them quickly in an oiled skillet. Season with salt and pepper. Place the fish on a plate along with the Brussels sprouts and the mango salsa. Garnish with lime wedges and cilantro and serve.

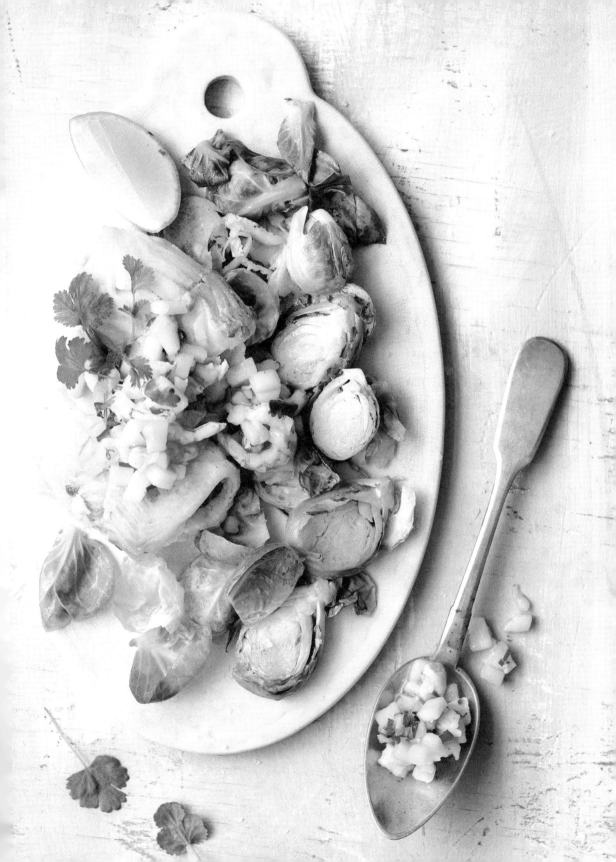

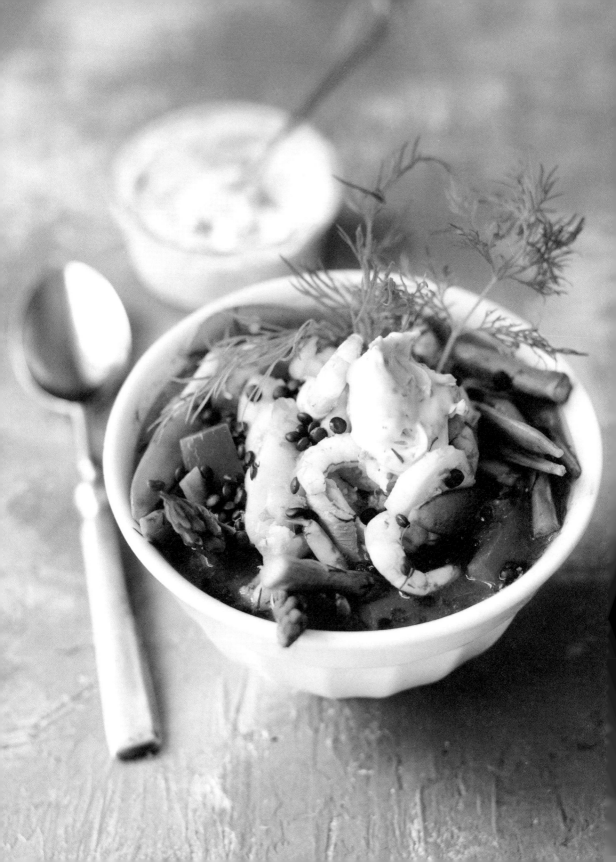

FISH SOUP

SERVES 4

1¼ lb (500 g) shrimp, in the shell

1 tbsp olive oil

⅘ cup (200 ml) white wine or water

1 fennel bulb

1 yellow onion

1–2 garlic cloves

1 tbsp butter

⅖ cup (100 ml) Le Puy or Beluga lentils

0.017 oz (½ g) saffron threads

1 red chili

1 tbsp liquid honey

14 oz (400 g) canned crushed tomatoes

1 tbsp fresh thyme, chopped

Salt and black pepper

14 oz (400 g) fresh or frozen cod fillets

7 oz (200 g) fresh green asparagus

5¼ oz (150 g) sugar snap peas

½ red bell pepper

½ yellow bell pepper

Fresh dill, for garnish

DILL MAYONNAISE

⅖ cup (100 ml) mayonnaise

3 tbsp chopped dill

Salt and white pepper

Peel the shrimp and transfer the shells to a skillet. Add the olive oil and fry the shells for a few minutes. Stir in the wine and let it all reduce for a few more minutes. Strain, and save the shrimp stock.

Clean and cut the fennel bulb in half. Remove the hard, inner core and slice the rest of the fennel into thin slivers. Slice the onion into thin slivers, and finely chop the garlic.

Heat the butter in a large saucepan and cook the fennel, onion, and garlic together with the lentils for a few minutes. Finely chop the chili. Stir in the saffron, chili, honey, shrimp stock, crushed tomatoes, and thyme. Let everything simmer a few minutes, and then season with salt and pepper.

Cut fish, asparagus, sugar snap peas, and bell peppers into bite-size chunks. Add them to the soup pot and simmer for about 5 minutes, or until the fish is cooked through. Add the shrimp.

Mix all the mayonnaise ingredients together in a bowl. Ladle the soup into bowls and top with dill mayonnaise and pinches of dill.

ULRIKA'S PERSIAN LAMB STEW

SERVES 6

2 yellow onions

4 garlic cloves

1–2 green or red chilies

3 tbsp butter

3¼–4½ lb (1½–2 kg) lamb stew meat

2 tbsp grated fresh ginger

Salt and black pepper

2 tbsp ground cardamom

1 tbsp ground cinnamon

2 tbsp curry powder

14 oz (400 g) canned crushed tomatoes

1¼ cup (300 ml) water

2 tbsp kecap manis

1 organic meat stock cube

3½ oz (100 g) dried prunes or apricots

2 cinnamon sticks

10 cardamom pods

1 bunch salad onions

1 bunch fresh cilantro (save some for topping)

FOR SERVING

⅘ cup (200 ml) Turkish yogurt

⅖ cup (100 ml) pistachios, chopped

Lemon wedges

Slice the onions into slivers, and finely chop the garlic and chilies. Heat the butter in a skillet and sauté the meat, onions, garlic, chilies, and ginger. Do this in several batches, while seasoning with salt, pepper, cardamom, cinnamon, and curry. Place everything in a large cast-iron stewpot or Dutch oven.

Stir in the crushed tomatoes, water, kecap manis, stock cube, dried prunes, cinnamon sticks, and cardamom pods. Chop the salad onions and cilantro, and add them to the stewpot. Let it all simmer, covered, for 1½–2 hours.

Taste and add extra seasoning if needed, and serve with yogurt, chopped cilantro, pistachios, and lemon wedges.

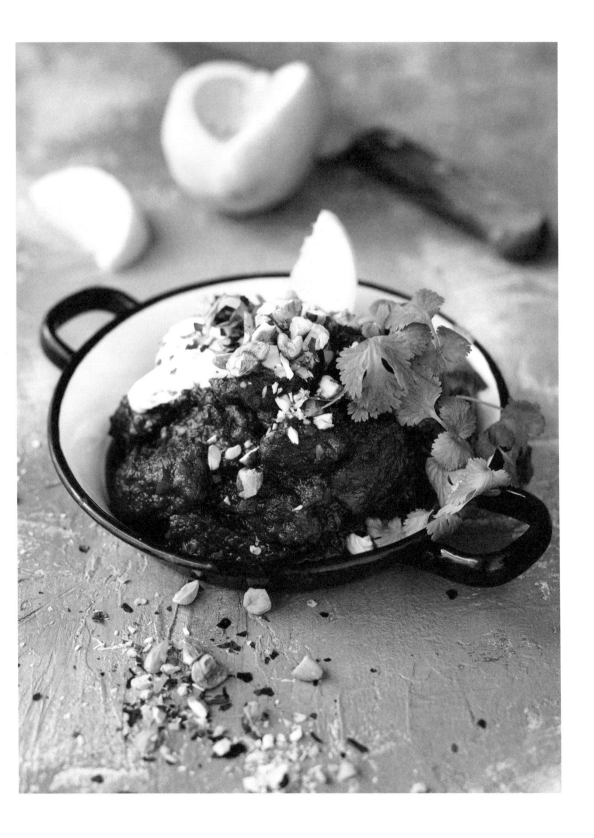

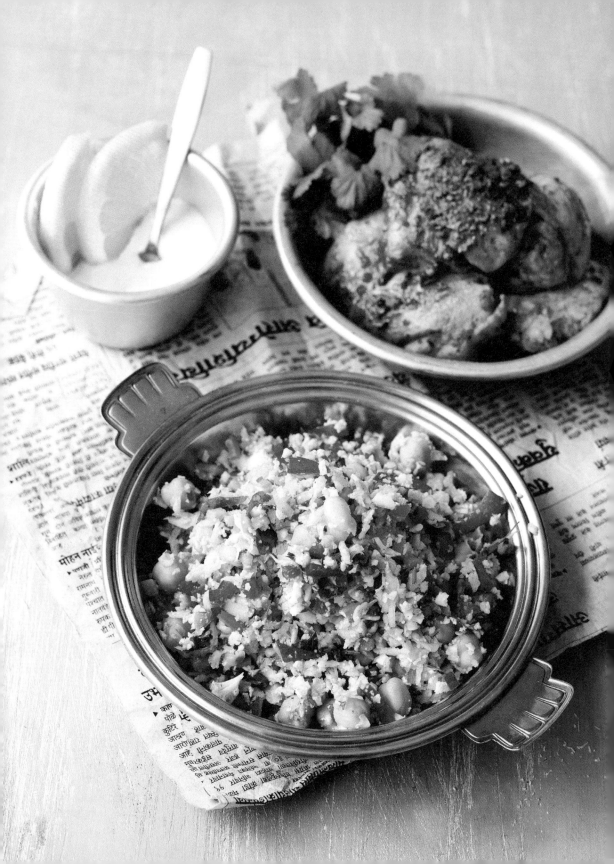

CAULIFLOWER RICE WITH CURRIED CHICKEN

SERVES 2

1 tsp butter

10½ oz (300 g) boneless chicken thighs

Salt and black pepper

1 tsp curry powder

⅛ tsp turmeric

½ tsp ground cumin

½ tbsp kecap manis

⅖ cup (100 ml) water

CAULIFLOWER RICE

½ head cauliflower

½ red onion

1 carrot

½ red bell pepper

½ tbsp olive oil

1 tsp curry powder

⅛ tsp turmeric

Juice from ½ lemon

Salt and black pepper

⅖ cup (100 ml) canned chickpeas

⅕ cup (50 ml) Italian parsley, finely chopped

Cooking yogurt*, for serving

Heat the butter in a skillet and sauté the chicken thighs for a few minutes. Season with salt, pepper, curry powder, turmeric, and cumin. Stir in the kecap manis and water, and let simmer for about 10 minutes or until the chicken is cooked through.

Meanwhile, prepare the cauliflower rice: Grate the cauliflower coarsely with a box grater. Finely chop the red onion, carrot, and bell pepper.

Saute everything for a couple of minutes in hot oil, and add curry powder, turmeric, lemon juice, salt, and pepper. Stir in the chickpeas and parsley. Serve with the chicken and yogurt.

*Cooking yogurt is a Swedish ingredient. Use 1 part yogurt to 2 parts sour cream.

GLUTEN-FREE TORTILLA WRAPS WITH CHICKEN AND PAPAYA

SERVES 4

½ small papaya

1 orange

1¼ lb (500 g) boneless chicken breast

½ tbsp olive oil

Salt and black pepper

1 tsp herb garden blend (store-bought)

Juice from ½ lemon

1 bag of lettuce

⅖ cup (100 ml) green peas

⅕ cup (50 ml) chopped pistachios

⅖ cup (100 ml) chopped chives

ORANGE DRESSING

Grated zest from 1 orange

⅘ cup (200 ml) cooking yogurt*

Salt and black pepper

1 tsp liquid honey

GLUTEN-FREE TORTILLAS

Makes 8 tortillas

5¼ oz (150 g) cornmeal

1 oz (30 g) psyllium husk

1 tsp baking powder

1 tsp salt

14 oz (400 ml) cold water

Start by making the tortillas: In a bowl, mix all the ingredients to make a smooth dough. Let it stand 15 minutes to let it rise.

Divide the dough into 8 pieces, and roll them out thinly on a work surface dusted with cornmeal. Fry the tortillas in a dry skillet until they have some color on both sides. Place the breads on top of one another and cover them with a kitchen towel to prevent them from drying out.

Mix all the ingredients for the orange dressing in a bowl and stir thoroughly. Set aside.

Slice the papaya. Remove the pith from the orange, and cut out nice-size wedges of the fruit.

Slice the chicken. Heat the oil in a skillet and brown the chicken all over. Season with salt, pepper, and herb garden blend. Stir in the lemon juice, and let the chicken simmer on low heat for about 20 minutes or until the meat is cooked through.

Put some lettuce, papaya and orange slices, chicken, and peas on each tortilla. Top with a dollop of orange dressing, some pistachios, and chives. Roll the tortilla up into a wrap, and enjoy.

*Cooking yogurt is a Swedish ingredient. Use 1 part yogurt to 2 parts sour cream

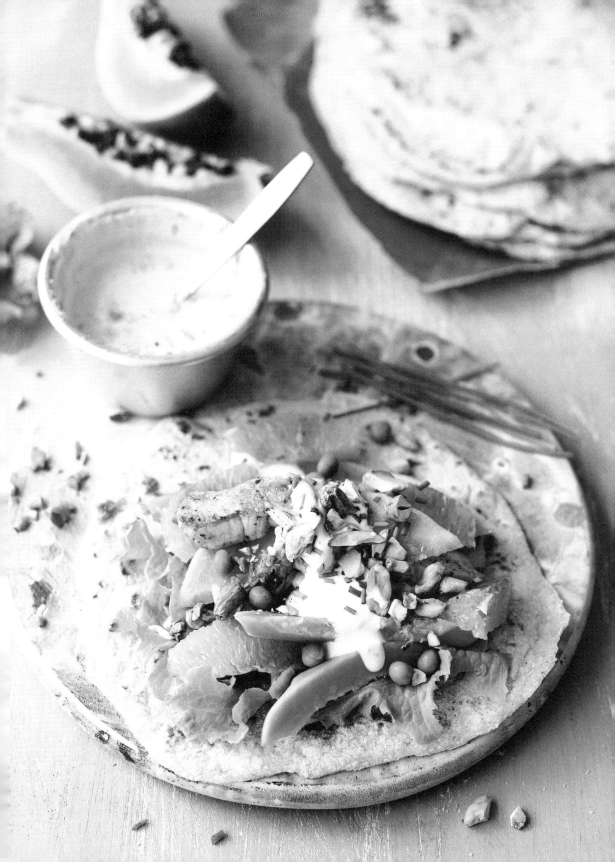

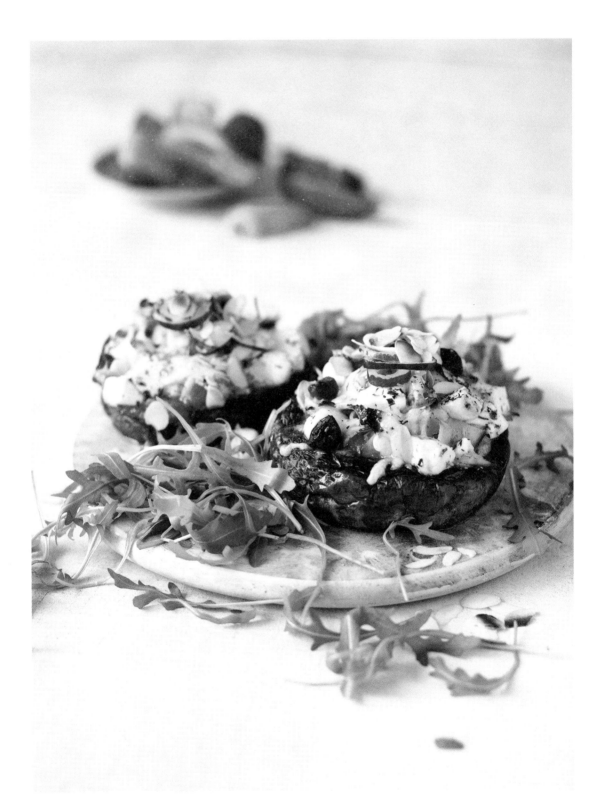

PORTABELLA MUSHROOM WITH AJVAR RELISH AND TURKEY BREAST

SERVES 2

2 large portabella
  mushrooms

3 tbsp ajvar relish

4 slices hot-smoked
  turkey breast

3½ oz (100 g) feta cheese

⅕ cup (50 ml) grated
  cheese (your choice)

½ red onion, sliced

2 tbsp black olives, sliced

2 tbsp flaked almonds

⅕ tsp herb garden blend
  (store-bought)

Arugula, for serving

Preheat the oven to 400°F (200°C). Put the mushrooms, upside down, onto a rimmed baking sheet, and spread ajvar relish on them. Place two slices of turkey on top of each mushroom, followed by the feta and grated cheese. Add red onion, olives, and flaked almonds to the mushrooms.

Sprinkle the mushrooms with herb garden blend, and bake for 20 minutes. Serve with arugula.

MEATBALLS WITH CAULIFLOWER RISOTTO

SERVES 2

1 small garlic clove

½ yellow onion

10½ oz (300 g) ground beef

2 tbsp chopped parsley

½ tsp dried garden herb blend (store-bought)

Salt and black pepper

½ tbsp olive oil, for frying

CAULIFLOWER RISOTTO

½ red onion

½ small garlic clove

6 mushrooms

½ tbsp olive oil

¼ head cauliflower

⅖ cup (100 ml) grated Parmesan cheese

1 tbsp chopped parsley

Salt and black pepper

FOR SERVING

⅘ cup (200 ml) arugula lettuce, ½ sliced red bell pepper, 2 slices of orange, sprigs of parsley, ajvar relish, aioli, and grated Parmesan cheese

Finely chop the garlic and yellow onion, and place them in a bowl. Add ground beef, parsley, garden herb blend, salt, and pepper, and mix thoroughly. Make meatballs. Heat the oil in a skillet and brown the meatballs on all sides for a few minutes.

Finely chop the red onion and garlic for the cauliflower risotto. Slice the mushrooms. Sauté everything in an oiled skillet for a few minutes. Grate the cauliflower finely with a box grater, and stir into the skillet. Sauté for a few minutes, and add the Parmesan and the parsley. Season with salt and pepper.

Put the arugula on plates, and layer the cauliflower risotto, meatballs, and bell pepper on top. Garnish with orange slices and parsley. Serve with ajvar relish, aioli, and Parmesan.

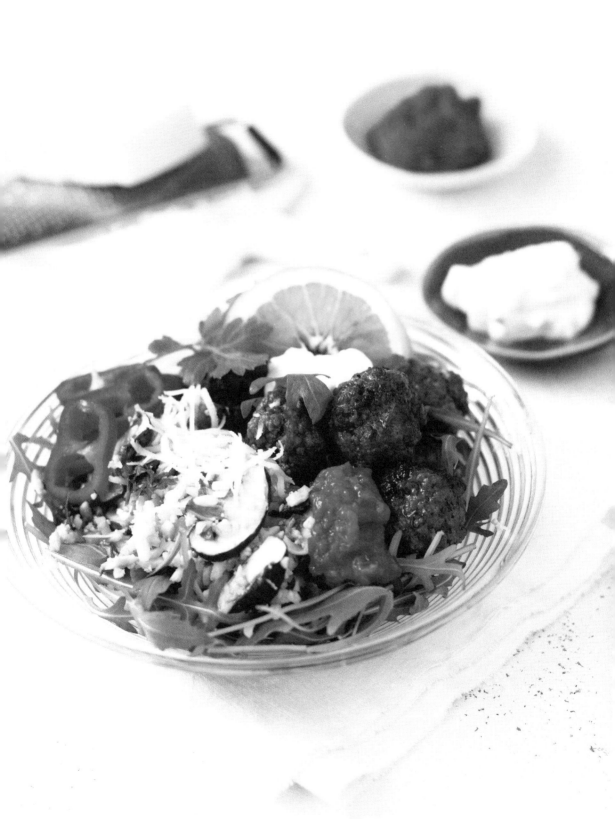

DESSERTS

Now and then it's nice to enjoy something sweet at the end of the meal. Healthy dessert recipes are always welcome, and here I'll share with you a few favorites of mine that I often make when I entertain—each one without gluten or refined white sugar!

Chocolate rounds with nuts and dried fruit 144 * Chocolate rounds with pomegranate 145 * Four delicious raw food balls 146 * Mango and raspberry sorbet with chocolate mousse 148 * Raw gooey cake 151 * Raw lemon cake with coconut and raspberries 152 * Stuffed melon 155

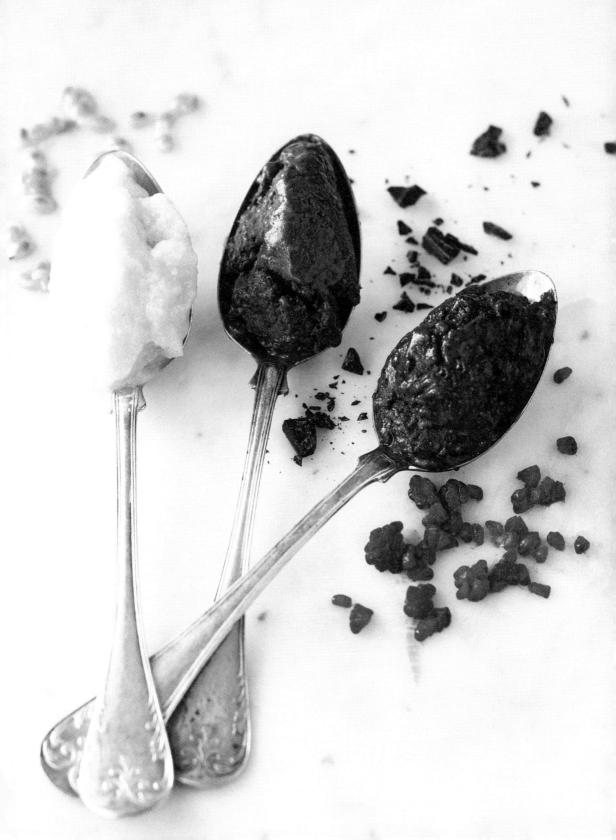

CHOCOLATE ROUNDS WITH NUTS AND DRIED FRUIT

MAKES 20 PIECES

5¼ oz (150 g) dark chocolate, 70% cocoa

⅘ cup (200 ml) mix of dried fruit and berries, nuts and seeds (such as cranberries, pine nuts, goji berries, dried fruit mix, pistachios, pumpkin seeds, hemp seeds)

Chop up the chocolate and melt it over a water bath. Place rounds of chocolate on a baking sheet or tray lined with parchment paper. Sprinkle the dried fruit, dried berries, nuts, and seeds over the top, and let the chocolate rounds chill in the refrigerator for 1 hour.

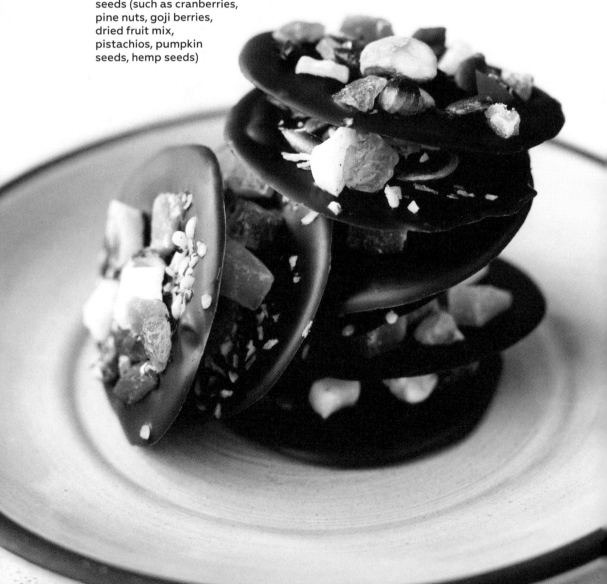

CHOCOLATE ROUNDS
WITH POMEGRANATE

MAKES 20 PIECES

5¼ oz (150 g) dark
   chocolate, 70% cocoa

Seeds from 1
   pomegranate

Chop up the chocolate and melt it over a water
bath. Place rounds of chocolate on a baking sheet
or tray lined with parchment paper.

Sprinkle pomegranate seeds on top, and let the
chocolate rounds chill in the refrigerator for 1 hour.

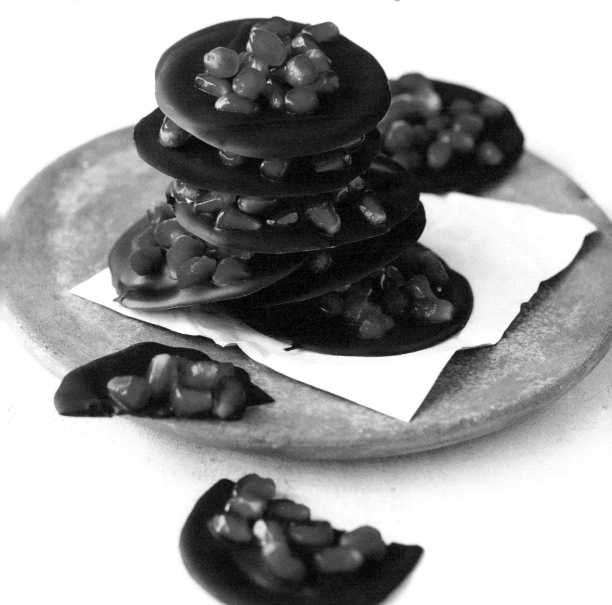

FOUR DELICIOUS RAW FOOD BALLS

These slightly healthier treats are perfect to have on hand when a sugar craving strikes. Go on, make a double batch—they freeze well.

CITRUS BALLS

MAKES 14

- 4⅔ cups (400 ml) almonds
- 2½ oz (75 ml) freshly-squeezed orange juice
- 3 dried dates, pits removed
- 1 tsp vanilla powder
- Grated peel from 2 oranges, for covering
- Grated peel from 3 lemons, for covering

In a food processor or blender, mix all the ingredients to make a paste. Form balls with the paste, and roll them in the orange and lemon peel to cover. Store the balls in the refrigerator or freezer.

CHOCOLATE BALLS

MAKES 14

- ⅘ cup (200 ml) almonds
- ⅘ cup (200 ml) walnuts
- ⅘ cup (200 ml) coconut flakes
- 5 dried dates, pits removed
- 4 tbsp cocoa
- Pinch of salt
- 2 to 3 tbsp water
- ⅖ cup (100 ml) cocoa, for covering

In a food processor or blender, mix almonds, walnuts, coconut flakes, dates, cocoa, and salt to make a paste, adding water until the paste has a workable consistency.

Form balls with the paste, and roll them in cocoa to cover. Store the balls in the refrigerator or freezer.

SPIRULINA BALLS

MAKES 14

- 1¼ cups cashews
- ⅖ cup (100 ml) pumpkin seeds
- 4 dried figs
- 2 tbsp spirulina powder
- 2 to 3 tbsp water
- ⅖ cup (100 ml) chopped pumpkin seeds, for covering

In a food processor or blender, mix all the ingredients except chopped pumpkin seeds to make a paste, adding water until the paste has a workable consistency. Form balls with the paste and roll them in the chopped pumpkin seeds to cover. Store the balls in the refrigerator or freezer.

RASPBERRY BALLS

MAKES 14

- ⅖ cup (100 ml) cashews
- ⅖ cup (100 ml) coconut flakes
- 3 dried apricots
- ⅖ cup (100 ml) frozen raspberries
- ⅕ tsp vanilla powder
- Lingonberry powder, for covering

In a food processor or blender, mix all the ingredients except the lingonberry powder to make a paste. Form the paste into balls and roll them in the lingonberry powder. Store the balls in the refrigerator or freezer.

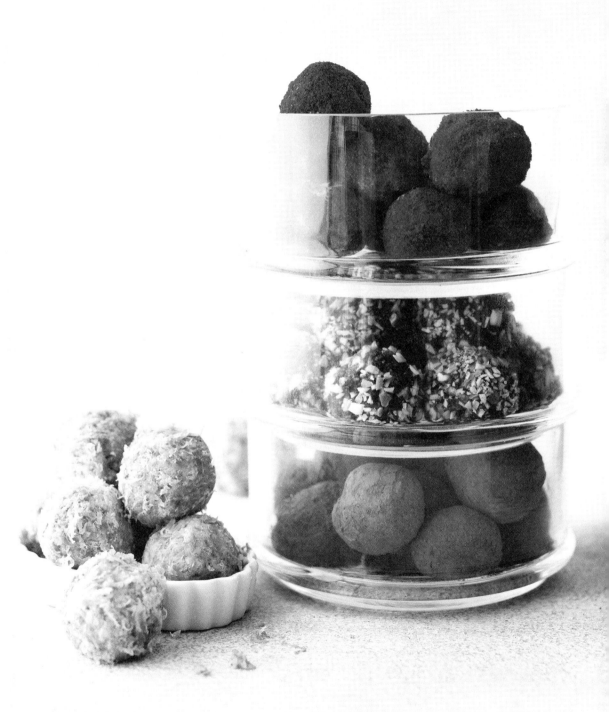

MANGO AND RASPBERRY SORBET WITH CHOCOLATE MOUSSE

RASPBERRY SORBET

7 oz (200 g) frozen raspberries

1 banana

2 tbsp coconut cream

MANGO SORBET

4½ oz (125 g) frozen diced mango

⅔ cup (100 ml) fresh-squeezed orange juice

Juice from ½ lime

CHOCOLATE MOUSSE

3 dried dates, pits removed

1 tbsp cocoa

½ avocado

1 frozen banana, sliced

TOPPING

Fresh red and/or black currants and raspberries

Process the different mixtures separately to smooth consistency in either a food processor or a blender.

Start with a bottom layer of raspberry sorbet, add a layer of mango sorbet, and finish with the chocolate mousse. Top with fresh berries, and serve immediately.

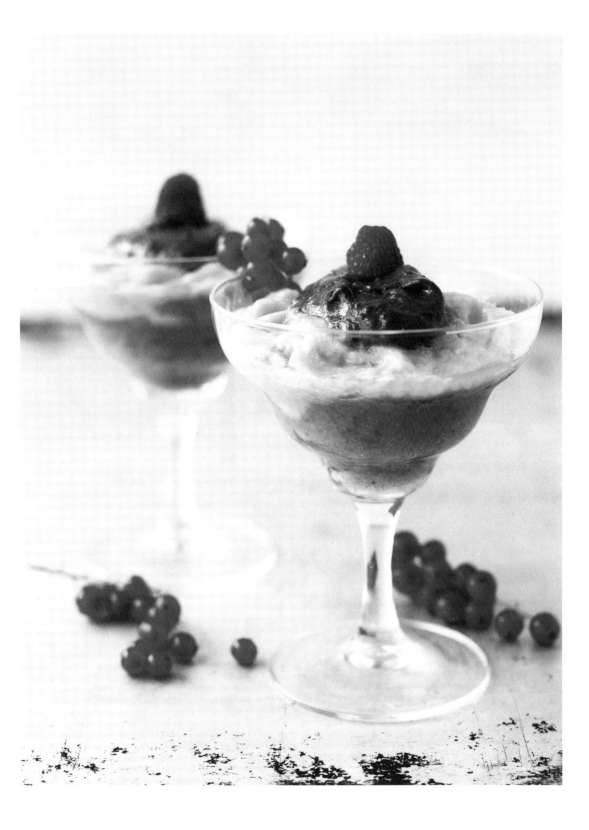

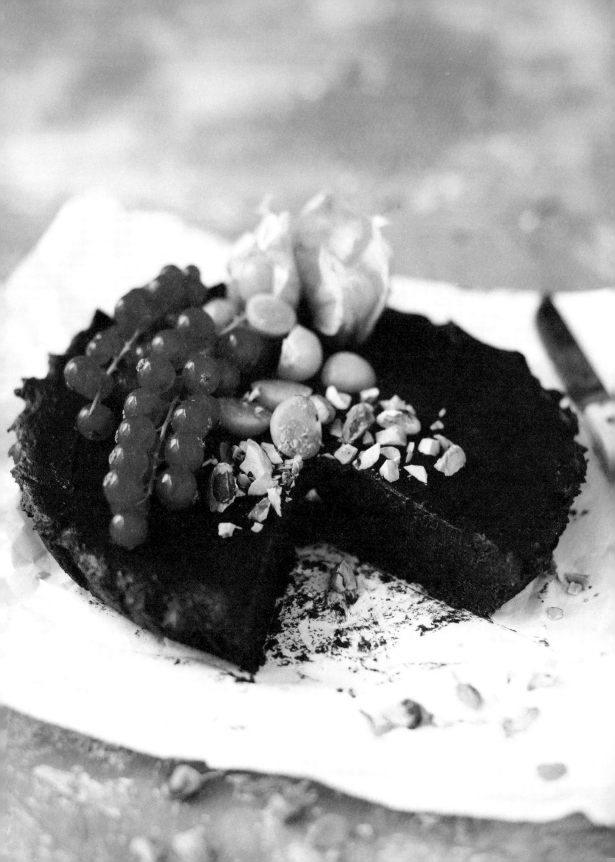

RAW GOOEY CAKE

BOTTOM LAYER

2⅓ cups (500 ml) walnuts

1½ cups (350 ml) dried
   dates, pits removed

1 avocado

Pinch of salt flakes

1 tsp grated orange peel

2 tsp vanilla powder

⅖ cup (100 ml) cocoa

CHOCOLATE CRÈME

3 avocados

Pinch of salt flakes

⅖ cup (100 ml) cocoa

⅖ cup (100 ml) agave
   syrup

TOPPING

⅕ cup (50 ml) chopped
   pistachios, fresh red
   and/or black currants,
   ground-cherries

For the bottom layer, chop the walnuts and dates coarsely in a food processor. Add the avocado flesh with the remaining ingredients, and mix to make a smooth paste.

Line an 8″ (20 cm) pie pan with removable edge (or a springform pan) with parchment paper. Pour the bottom layer evenly into the pie pan.

Place the avocado flesh and other ingredients for the chocolate crème in a food processor and process to make a smooth cream. Spread this cream over the bottom layer, and let chill in the refrigerator for 2–3 hours. Garnish the cake with pistachios, red and/or black currants, and ground cherries.

RAW LEMON CAKE WITH COCONUT AND RASPBERRIES

SERVES 8

BOTTOM LAYER

⅖ cup (100 ml) dried
  dates, pits removed

⅖ cup (100 ml) walnuts

Pinch of salt

FILLING

1½ cups (350 ml) coconut
  flakes

Grated peel of 2 lemons

⅖ cup (100 ml) freshly-
  squeezed lemon juice

3 tbsp coconut oil

4 tbsp agave syrup

½ tsp vanilla powder

½ tsp turmeric

Pinch of salt

TOPPING

⅗ cup (150 ml) fresh
  raspberries

Grated lemon peel

2 tbsp coconut flakes

In a food processor or blender, mix the ingredients for the bottom layer to make a smooth paste. Line a 6¼-inch (16 cm) pie pan with removable edge (or a springform pan) with parchment paper. Press the paste evenly into the pie pan.

In a blender or food processor, process the coconut flakes for the filling to make coconut butter—this will take about 5 minutes. Add in the remaining ingredients and mix.

Spread the filling over the bottom layer, and let the cake chill in the refrigerator for at least one hour. Garnish the cake with raspberries, lemon zest, and coconut flakes.

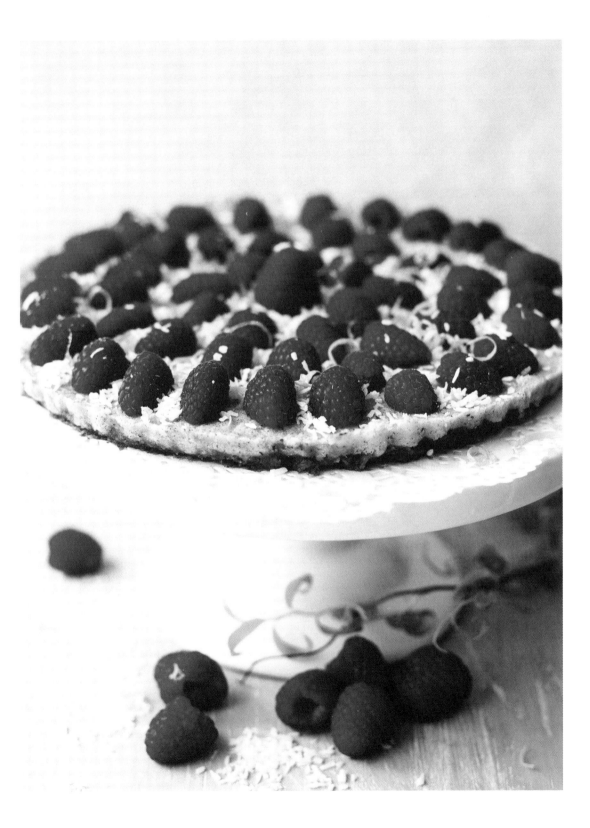

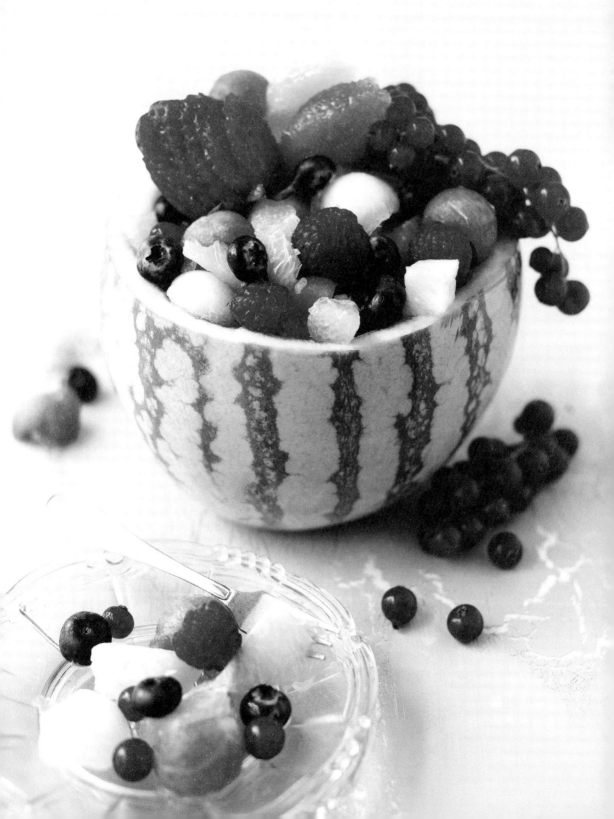

Fruit in all its simplicity is wonderfully delicious, but when prepared like this, it's even better. Serve it with some vanilla yogurt, if you like.

STUFFED MELON

SERVES 2

1 small watermelon

¼ honeydew melon

¼ fresh pineapple

1 grapefruit

1 orange

⅖ cup (100 ml) fresh
  blueberries and
  raspberries

TOPPING

2 sliced strawberries

2 bunches red and/or
  black currants

Cut the watermelon across the middle. Scoop out the watermelon and the honeydew with an ice cream scoop, and place the scooped-out watermelon and melon flesh in a bowl.

Cut the pineapple into small chunks. Peel the grapefruit and orange with a very sharp knife, and cut out fine segments of the fruit, leaving the pith behind. Cut the segments into chunks. Mix all the fruit in the bowl, along with the blueberries and raspberries. Divide the chopped fruit between the two scooped-out halves of watermelon, and garnish with the strawberries and bunches of red and/ or black currants.

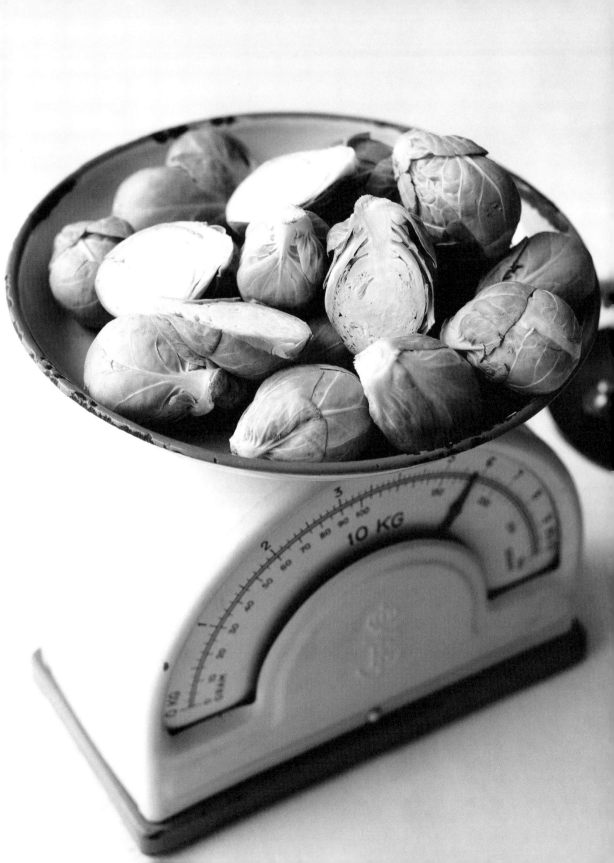

A TWO-WEEK DIET PLAN

Would you like some help starting eating foods that are healthy and beneficial to hormonal balance? If so, here is a practical two-week diet plan that will give you a jump-start with the right foods, and that will facilitate planning ahead.

The diet plan is based on low-carbohydrate foods that use natural ingredients, thus providing you with energy and making you feel satiated. You can substitute recipe ingredients for similar alternatives, and you can add in all the herbs and spices you like. Some recipes make two servings, so that the second serving can become your lunch or dinner some other day. If you're invited to a party or eating in a restaurant, try to select options that seem in line with the plan's menu.

Always start your day with some lemon water (see p. 55) or a shot of ginger and lime (see p. 54). Continue to drink plenty of water throughout the day, preferably about 2 quarts (2 liters), and feel free to add herb tea or green tea to this, too.

This diet plan is put together to help you maintain hormonal balance, to provide a boost to your metabolism, to refresh your awareness of portion sizes, and to make you lose about 6½ pounds (3 kg) in two weeks. You'll be consuming a variable number of calories—between 500 to 2,000—to give your metabolism a push. That means that on some days you'll eat a little less, and other days a bit more. You may change the sequence of "full days," and you can switch around between lunch and dinner, but do not replace one day's meal with a meal from different day.

You can still follow the plan even if you're not looking to lose weight, but want to modify your diet to balance out your hormones to help you feel better mentally and physically. In that case, you can eat slightly larger portions and a healthy snack, like seed buns or a green smoothie.

DAY	BREAKFAST	LUNCH	DINNER
Monday (1,115 calories)	1 flaxseed bun, p. 73 with 1 tsp butter, cheese and bell pepper (290 calories)	Zucchini pasta with pesto, p. 78 (500 calories)	Cod roulades with mango salsa, p. 128 (325 calories)
Tuesday (859 calories)	Green smoothie with basil, p. 64 (204 calories)	Spinach soup with avocado and peas, p. 107 (184 calories)	Italian chicken pot, p. 124 (471 calories)
Wednesday (1,591 calories)	5 fl oz (150 ml) yogurt or oat milk yogurt with 3⅓ fl oz (100 ml) crunchy granola, p. 62 (278 calories)	Omelet wrap with choice of filling, p. 102 (approx. 500 calories)	Mozzarella salad with Chioggia beets, p. 82 (813 calories)
Thursday (655 calories)	Black coffee, green tea, or herb tea	Spinach soup with avocado and peas (leftovers, 184 calories)	Italian chicken pot (leftovers, 471 calories)
Friday (1,592 calories)	Oat porridge "to go," p. 61 (your choice, approx. 500 calories)	Swedish salad, p. 93 (552 calories)	Meatloaf with oven-roasted tomatoes, p. 122 (540 calories)
Saturday (1,933 calories)	Smoothie bowl, p. 66 (your choice, 500 calories)	Marinated beets with chèvre gratin, p. 85 (425 calories)	Fish soup, p. 131 (598 calories); Raw lemon cake with coconut and raspberries, p. 152 (200 calories); 2 glasses of wine (210 calories)
Sunday (1,358 calories)	Omelet with pear, feta, and raspberries, p. 70 (393 calories)	Meatloaf with oven-roasted tomatoes (leftovers, 540 calories)	Marinated beets with chèvre gratin, p. 85 (leftovers, 425 calories)

DAY	BREAKFAST	LUNCH	DINNER
Monday (1,490 calories)	Chia porridge with mango and orange, p. 57 (375 calories)	Gluten-free tortilla wraps with chicken and papaya, p. 136 (500 calories)	Meatballs with cauliflower risotto, p. 140 (615 calories)
Tuesday (822 calories)	Green smoothie with basil, p. 64 (204 calories)	Raw food salad, p. 98 (378 calories)	Carrot soup with ginger and chicken bacon, p. 105 (240 calories)
Wednesday (1,578 calories)	5 fl oz (150 ml) yogurt or oat yogurt with 3⅓ fl oz (100 ml) crunchy granola, p. 62 (278 calories)	Gluten-free tortilla wraps with chicken and papaya (leftovers, 500 calories)	Fruity rice stir-fry with seared salmon and aioli, p. 116 (800 calories)
Thursday (548 calories)	Black coffee, green tea, or herb tea	Carrot soup with ginger and chicken bacon (leftovers, 240 calories)	Melon salad with chèvre and avocado, p. 81 (308 calories)
Friday (1,775 calories)	Oat porridge "to go," p. 61 (your choice, approx. 500 calories)	Fruity rice stir-fry with seared salmon and aioli (leftovers, 800 calories)	Chicken wrapped in rice paper, p. 86 (475 calories)
Saturday (1,906 calories)	Scrambled eggs with brie cheese, p. 69 (466 calories)	Chicken wrapped in rice paper (leftovers, 475 calories)	Portabella mushroom with ajvar relish and turkey breast, p. 139 (390 calories); Mango and raspberry sorbet with chocolate mousse, p. 148 (365 calories); 2 glasses of wine (210 calories)
Sunday (1,210 calories)	1 flaxseed bun, p. 73 with 1 tsp butter, cheese and bell pepper (250 calories)	Omelet wrap with choice of filling, p. 102 (approx. 500 calories)	Asian salmon soup with seagrass noodles, p. 110 (460 calories)

GLOSSARY

Adrenaline: Stress hormone secreted by the adrenal glands that stimulates our "fight or flight" reflex in case of perceived danger.

Amenorrhea: The absence of menstruation; a missed period.

Amino acids: The body's building blocks—proteins—are made up of amino acids. When you eat protein, it's broken down into amino acids in the digestive system. Tyrosine and tryptophan are two examples of amino acids. They are needed to produce neurotransmitters in the body.

Antioxidants: An umbrella term for substances primarily found in fruits and vegetables that protect us from free radicals (molecules that can cause damage in our bodies on a cellular level).

Biochemistry: The branch of science that deals with the chemistry of all living things (including us humans). A living cell is made up of many different molecules, which all react with each other by different chemical processes.

Bioidentical hormones: As opposed to synthetically made hormones, bioidentical hormones have the same molecular structure as the hormones made by the body. That's why the body "recognizes" these hormones and works with them the same way it would with hormones produced by your ovaries.

Brain fog: Impaired cognitive function where concentration, memory, and motivation are affected. You can feel disconnect and have trouble finding the right word.

CBT (cognitive behavioral therapy): A method of psychotherapeutic treatment in which the aim is to change thought, emotional, and behavioral patterns that negatively affect the individual.

Cortisol: A hormone that is produced by the adrenal glands that regulates stress and immune response.

DHA: Docosahexaenoic acid is an essential fatty acid from the omega-3 family. DHA contributes, among other things, to the normal functioning of the brain. "Essential" means that your body depends on this fatty acid but cannot produce it on its own; you need to obtain it through your diet, i.e., the food you eat.

Dysbiosis (dysbacterieosis): The imbalance between good and bad microorganisms in the gut flora.

Enzymes: Digestive enzymes are produced in different areas in the digestive system and are needed for the breakdown of food. Minerals, vitamins, or fats can't be absorbed by the colon if they are not broken down by enzymes.

EPA: Eicosapentaenoic acid is an essential fatty acid belonging to the omega-3 family. EPA has the same function as DHA (see previous). "Essential" means that your body depends on this fatty acid but cannot produce it on its own; you need to obtain it through your diet, i.e., the food you eat.

Estrogen: A hormone primarily considered a female sex hormone. It exists in both men and women, but in much larger amounts in women. A woman's ovaries secrete three types of estrogen: estradiol, estrone, and estriol.

Estrogen dominance: An imbalance between progesterone and estrogen in which the level of progesterone is too low compared to the level of estrogen.

GMO: A genetically modified organism is one whose genes have been changed, but not in a natural way, such as with mating or cross-pollination.

Hormone receptors: These are proteins situated on the surface of certain cells throughout the body, including breast cells. These receptor proteins receive messages from hormones in the blood, at which point they tell the cells what to do. If the correct substance fits the receptor, the receptor is activated, and a specific activity begins in the cell.

Indole-3-carbinol: A natural substance found in cruciferous vegetables (Brussels sprouts and cauliflower, for instance) that is important in the liver's ability to neutralize toxins. It also helps the body get rid of used estrogen.

Insulin resistance: Insulin helps the cells' uptake of glucose (energy) from the blood. However, with excessive consumption of sugar and quick carbohydrates, this system can become worn out. The insulin's effect is impaired, making excess glucose stay in the blood, which elevates blood sugar.

Leaky gut syndrome (intestinal hyper-permeability): There are small holes in the lining of the small intestine that allow nutrients to pass through to the bloodstream. If inflammation is present, the holes become enlarged, which lets colon bacteria, fungus, undigested food, and waste products pass through into the bloodstream. Over the long term this can cause autoimmune illness and inflammation in the body.

Menopause ("change of life"): A hormonal phase that lasts about a year after menstruation has ceased.

Nutritional medicine: Knowledge on how diet, vitamins, minerals, amino acids, fatty acids, enzymes, probiotics, and antioxidants affect the body's anatomy, physiology, and psychology.

PCOS (polycystic ovarian syndrome): A condition in which one or both ovaries are filled with fluid-packed blisters called cysts. They are detectable by ultrasound exam of the ovaries.

Perimenopause: The hormonal phase that can last between one and ten years before menstruation stops.

PMS (premenstrual syndrome): Mood swings and other problems that occur one or two weeks prior to menstruation. The symptoms disappear quickly once the period starts.

Postmenopausal: A hormonal phase following menopause. Continues until the end of life.

Prebiotics: Complex carbohydrates that are not broken down by the digestive system but reach the colon in their original form. Prebiotics feed the probiotic bacteria.

Probiotics: Lactic acid bacteria that are vital for gut and intestinal health, immune response, and the breakdown of nutrients in the colon. A deficiency in lactic acid affects the immune system, hormones, and body weight.

Progesterone (yellow body hormone): A sex hormone that is produced in the corpus luteum in the ovaries after ovulation.

Serotonin: Serotonin is a neurotransmitter that provides a sense of well-being and happiness. Counteracts anxiety and depression.

Testosterone: A sex hormone that is often considered a male sex hormone. It exists in both men and women, but in much larger amounts in men. The ovaries and adrenal glands produce testosterone in women, whereas the testicles and adrenal glands produce testosterone in men.

Toxins: Poisonous substances that can cause illness and damage to the body.

Tryptophan: An essential amino acid that we obtain through the diet. Tryptophan is vital to the production of body proteins, serotonin, and melatonin.

INDEX

5-methyltetrahydrofolate **28**
acetylcholine **27**
acetylsalicylic acid **28**
adrenaline **10**
acne **33, 36**
alcohol **14, 21, 46**
alcoholism **28**
amenorrhea
amino acids **9, 14, 23, 27**
amylase **38**
anger **16, 18**
antibiotics **34, 35, 36**
anti-inflammatory food **31**
anti-inflammatory medications
    30
antioxidants **26, 31**
anxiety **8, 23, 24, 25, 41, 42**
apathy **17, 18, 26, 32**
appetite, lack of **29**
artificial colorants **46**
artificial sweeteners **41**
asthma **30, 34**
B9 (Folic acid) **27, 28, 38, 40**
B vitamins **27**
belching **38**
beta-glucuronidase **35**
bifidobacteria **35**
bioidentical estrogen **42**
bioidentical progesterone **42**
bioidentical hormones,
    replacement **18, 41**
biorhythm, daily **18**
bloated abdomen **38**
bloating **36, 38**
blood clots **41**
blood glucose **19, 20, 22, 27, 31,
    32, 45**
blood glucose drop **32**
blood sugar crash **24**
brain chemistry **19**
brain fog **17, 23, 24, 32, 36**
brain tissue **21**
breakouts **34**
breast cancer **41, 42**
breathing exercises **40**
breathlessness **26**
C-reactive protein (CRP) **31**
calming **12**
cancer **29, 20**
cancer, uterine **42**

carbohydrates **14, 20, 23, 32**
carbohydrates, slow-release
    24, 33
carbohydrates, quick-acting **22,
    24, 32**
cardiologist **10**
cardiovascular disease **29, 30, 41**
casein **30**
CBT (cognitive behavioral
    therapy) **40**
change of life **17**
cholesterol **21, 41**
cobalamine, see also vitamin
    B12 **28**
concentrate, ability to **19, 20, 21,
    25, 26**
confusion **25, 28**
constipation **24, 34, 36**
contraceptive coil **18**
contraceptive pills **9, 21, 28, 35**
cortisol **10, 19, 31**
cravings, sweets **24**
dairy products **30, 45**
dementia **30**
diabetes **30, 31**
diarrhea **34, 36**
dietary supplements **14, 21,
    40, 48**
dieting **14**
diets **23**
digestive function **20**
digestive enzymes **38**
dizziness, see also vertigo **32**
dysbiosis **35**
docosahexaenoic acid (DHA)
    21, 22
dopamine **11, 13, 14, 20, 23, 26, 27**
eikosapentaenoic acid (EPA)
    21, 22
enterococcus **35**
environmental allergens **30**
Escherichia coli (E. coli) **35**
essential amino acids **21**
estradiol **11**
estriol **11**
estrogen **10, 11, 13, 15, 17, 21, 24,
    35, 39**
estrogen, blocking of **32**
estrogen dominance **17, 36**
estrogen receptors **19, 32, 33**

estrone **11**
enzymes **38**
enzyme deficiency **38**
exercise **21**
fat **20, 21**
fatigue **16, 19, 26, 27, 32, 34**
fatty acids **21**
feeling guilty **8**
fermented food **25, 37**
fiber **24**
fibromyalgia **29**
fish oil **25**
fluid balance **17**
focus **21**
follicle-stimulating hormone
    (FSH) **18**
folic acid (B9) **14, 28**
folic acid, lack of **28**
food allergies **30, 31, 34**
food, breakdown **34**
food intolerance **30, 31**
free radicals **26**
functional medicine **9, 31**
fungal infections **36**
GABA **11, 12, 14, 20**
GMO (genetically modified orga-
    nisms) **30**
gastric acid, see also hydrochlo-
    ric acid **38**
gastric reflux **38**
gastritis **30**
glutamate **24**
gluten **24**
glucose **23, 24, 27, 32**
good gut bacteria **31**
gut flora **20, 35**
hair loss **26**
hallucinations **29**
Hashimoto's thyroiditis **34**
headache **15, 26**
hormonal disturbances **32, 33**
hormonal imbalance **9**
hormone receptors **19**
hot flashes **11, 16, 17, 32**
hydrochloric acid **38**
IBD (Irritable Bowel Disease) **30**
IBS (Irritable Bowel Syndrome)
    9, 30
immune system **29, 30, 34**
indole-3-carbinol **37, 44**

infectious diseases **29**
infertility **33, 36**
inflamed brain **24**
inflamed gut **24**
inflammation **17, 19, 20, 22, 25, 30, 31, 32, 44, 45**
insulin **10, 19, 24, 32, 46**
insulin resistance **30, 31, 32, 33, 44**
insulin sensitivity **22**
intrinsic factor (IF) **29, 38**
iron **25, 26**
iron deficiency **17, 26, 36**
irritability **15, 16, 18, 19, 25, 26, 27**
lactobacilli **35**
lactose **30**
leaky gut, *see also* permeability of the intestines **25, 30**
learning **21, 26**
lethargy **27**
libido **18**
lipase **38**
logical thinking **26**
magnesium **14, 25**
mania **29**
medications **21**
meditation **19, 40**
melatonin **27**
memory **19, 21, 23, 25, 26, 27**
memory lapses **28**
menopause **8, 10, 15, 17, 18**
menstrual pain **25**
menstruation **15, 16, 17, 18**
mental inertia **27**
mindfulness **19, 40**
minerals **14, 20, 24, 25**
muscle aches **25**
muscle growth **22**
muscle weakness **29**
night sweats **16**
nerve cells **12**
nerve impulse **12**
nervous system **26, 28**
nervousness **26**
nervousness **8, 14, 15, 16, 18, 23, 24, 25, 27, 41, 42**
neurochemistry **9**
neurotransmitters **9, 12, 13, 14, 15, 19, 20, 21, 23, 25, 26**
noradrenalin **13, 20, 23**

nutritional deficiencies **9, 48**
nutritional medicine **9**
monounsaturated fats **31**
mood swings **18, 19, 26, 28**
obesity **30**
omega-3 fatty acids **21, 22, 40**
omega-6 fatty acids **22**
osteoarthritis **34**
osteoporosis **10, 29**
overweight **29, 30, 35**
ovulation **11, 16, 39**
PCOS (polycystic ovary syndrome) **33**
PMS (premenstrual syndrome) **8, 10, 11, 15, 16, 18, 25, 36**
pain **34**
palpitations **17, 26**
pancreas **32**
paranoia **29**
parasites **31**
perimenopause **8, 10, 16, 18, 26, 41, 43**
permeability of the intestines, *see also* leaky gut **34**
physical training **16**
pituitary gland **10, 39**
plaque, development of **11, 41**
postmenopausal **17, 18**
pregnancy **11, 16**
probiotics **25, 35**
progesterone **10, 11, 15, 16, 17, 19, 21, 39**
protease **38**
protein **20, 21, 22, 23**
red blood cells **28**
rest **21**
restlessness **14**
rheumatoid arthritis **34**
selenium **25, 26**
serotonin **11, 12, 13, 14, 20, 23, 26, 27**
serotonin receptors **11**
sleep **8, 12, 19, 23**
sleeping problems **11, 17, 18, 19, 20, 23, 26**
soothing
starch **22**
streptococcus **35**
stress **10, 11, 14, 15, 20, 21, 25, 27, 30, 31, 38, 39**

stress hormones **34**
stroke **30**
sugar **22**
sugar kick **24**
synapses **12**
synthetic hormones **41**
teenage years **15**
testosterone **10, 33, 39**
thyroid hormones **10, 17, 26, 36**
tyrosine **23**
thyroxine (T4) **10**
tingling sensation **29**
toxins **34, 35**
transfats **46**
triiodothyronine (T3) **10**
tryptophan **14, 23**
vagina **11**
vegan diets **21**
vegetarian diets **21**
vertigo, *see also* dizziness **32**

vitamin A **27**
vitamin B **27**
vitamin B1 (thiamine) **27**
vitamin B3 (niacin) **27**
vitamin B6 (pyridoxine) **14, 27, 40**
vitamin B12, *see also* cobalamine **27, 28, 38, 40**
vitamin C **27**
vitamin D **14**
vitamin D **25, 27, 29**
vitamin E **27**
vitamin K **27**
vitamins **9, 14, 20, 24, 27, 31**
weepiness **17, 18**
weight gain **17, 18, 19, 22, 31, 35, 44**
weight loss **24**
wholesome gut bacteria **19, 24, 31, 34**
wholesome lactic acid bacteria **34**
winter depression **29**
yellow body hormone, *see also* progesterone
yoga **19, 40**
zinc **25, 26**

SOURCES

ABOUT HORMONES

Abramovitz E S, Baker A H, Fleischer S F, "Onset of depressive psychiatric crises and the menstrual cycle." *American Journal of Psychiatry*, April 1982;139(4):475–478.

Bethea C L, Pecins-Thompson M, Schutzer W, Gundlah C, Lu Z, "Ovarian steroids and serotonin neural function." *Molecular Neurobiology*, 1998;18:87–122.

Blum I, Lerman M, Misrachi I, Nordenberg Y, Grosskopf I, Weizman A, Levy-Schiff R, Sulkes J, Vered Y, "Lack of plasma norepinephrine cyclicity, increased etradiol during the follicular phase, and of progesterone and gonadotrophins at ovulation in women with premenstrual syndrome." *Neuropsychobiology*, 2004;50(1):10–14.

Brinton R D, Thompson R F, Foy M R, Baudry M, Wang J, Finch C E, Morgan T E, Pike C J, Mack W J, Stanczyk F Z, Nilsen J, "Progesterone receptors: form and function in brain." *Front Neuroendocrinology*, May 2008;29(2):313–339. E-pub, 23 February 2008.

De Novaes Soares C, "Efficacy of estradiol for the treatment of depressive disorders in perimenopausal women: a double blind randomized placebo controlled trial." *Archives of General Psychiatry*, June 2001;58(6):529–534.

Joffe H, Cohen L S, "Estrogen, serotonin, and mood disturbance: where is the therapeutic bridge?" *Biological Psychiatry*, November 1988;44(9):798–811.

Österlund, M, Hurd Y, "Estrogen receptors in the human forebrain and the relation to neuropsychiatry disorders." *Progressive Neurobiology*, 2001;64:251–267.

Rybaczyk L A, Bahaw M J, Pathak D R, Moody S M, Gilcers R M, Holzshu D L, "An overlooked connection: serotonergic medication of estrogen-related physiology and pathology." *BMC Women's Health*, 20 December 2005;5:12.

Small G W, "Estrogen effects on the brain." *Journal of Gender-specific Medicine*, 1998;1:23–27.

FOOD—THE BUILDING BLOCKS FOR HORMONES AND A BRAIN IN BALANCE

Bruinsma K A, Taren D L, "Dieting, essential fatty acid intake, and depression." *Nutrition Review*, April 2000;58(4):98–108.

Facchinetti F, et al, "Oral magnesium successfully relieves premenstrual mood changes." *Obstetric and Gynecology*, August 1991;78:177–181.

Fontani G, Corradeshi F, Felici A, Alfatti F, Miglorini S, Lodi L, "Cognitive and physiological effects of omega-3 polyunsaturated fatty acid supplementation in healthy subjects." *European Journal of Clinical Investigation*, November 2005;35(11):691–699.

AVOID INFLAMMATION

Anisman H, Merali Z, "Cytokines, stress, and depressive illness." *Brain, Behavior, and Immunity*, 2002;16:513–524. doi:10.1016/S0880-1591(02)00009-0.

Slavich G M, Irwin M R, "From Stress to Inflammation and Major Depressive Disorder: A Social Signal Transduction Theory of Depression." *Psychological Bulletin*, May 2014;140(3):774–815.

BALANCE YOUR BLOOD GLUCOSE

Dunaif A, Givens J R, Haseltine F, Merriam G R (eds), "The Polycystic Ovary Syndrome". *Blackwell Scientific*, 1992.

Eckel R H, "Insulin resistance: an adaptation for weight maintenance." *The Lancet*, Volume 340, Issue 8833, 12 December 1992;1452–1453.

Franks S, "Polycystic ovary syndrome." *The New England Journal of Medicine*, 1995;333:853–861.

KEEP YOUR GUT HAPPY

Angelakis E, Armougom F, Million M, Raoult D, "The relationship between gut microbiota and weight gain in humans." *Future Microbiology*, Vol. 7, No. 1, January 2012;91–109. DOI10.221/fmb.11.142 (doi:10.221/fmb.11.142).

Colea C B, Fullera R, Cartera S M, "Effect of Probiotic Supplements of Lactobacillus acidophilus and Bifidobacterium adolescentis 2204 on β-glueosidase and β-glueuronidase Activity in the Lower Gut of Rats Associated with a Human Faecal Flora." *Microbial Ecology in Health and Disease*, Volume 2, Issue 3, 1989;223–225.

Rodrigues D, Rocha-Santos T A P, Pereira C I, Gomes A M, Malcata F X, Freitas A C, "The potential effect of FOS and inulin upon probiotic bacterium performance in curdled milk matrices." *Food Sci Technol*, 2011.

Rossi M, Corradini C, Amaretti A, Nicolini M, Pompei A, Zanoni S, Matteuzzi, D, "Fermentation of Fructooligosaccharides and Inulin by Bifidobacteria: a Comparative Study of Pure and Fecal Cultures." *Applied and Environmental Microbiology*, 2005.

LOWER YOUR STRESS

Berga S L, Loucks T L, "Stress Induced Anovulation". Emory University School of Medicine, 2007.

Scott, E, "The Benefits of Yoga for Stress Management." The New York Times Company, 6 Feb 2012.

Turakitwanakan W, Mekseepralard C, Busarakumtragut P, "Effects of mindfulness meditation on serum cortisol of medical students." *J Med Assoc Thai*, 2013.

BIOIDENTICAL HORMONES

Collins J A, Blake J M, Crosignani P G, "Breast cancer incidence in women with a history of progesterone deficiency." *Human Reproduction Update*, Nov-Dec 2005;(6):545–560.

Darj E, Nilsson S, Axelsson O, Hellberg D, "Clinical and endometrial effects of oestradio [sic] and progesterone in post-menopausal women." *Maturitas*, June 1991;13(2):109–15.

Ettinger B, "Reduced mortality associated with long-term post-menopausal estrogen therapy." *Obstetrics and Gynecology*, January 1996;87(1): 6–12.

Fitzpatrick L A, et al: "Comparison of regimens containing oral micronized progesterone of medroxyprogesterone acetate on quality of life in postmenopausal women: a cross-sectional survey." *Journal of Women's Health Gender Based Medicine*, May 2000;9(4):381–387.

Fournier A, Berrino F, Clavel-Chapelon F, "Unequal risks for breast cancer associated with different hormone replacement therapies: results from the E3N cohort study." *Breast Cancer Research and Treatment*, January 2008;107(1):103–111.

Goletiani N V, Keith D R, and Gorsky S J, "Progesterone: review of safety for clinical studies." *Exp Clin Psychopharmacol*, 2007;15:427–444.

Gompel A, "Micronized progesterone and its impact on the endometrium and breast vs. progestogens". *Climacteric*, 2012;15:18–25

L'Hermite M, "HRT optimization, using transdermal estradiol plus micronized progesterone a safer HRT." *Climacteric*, 2013;16:44–53.

Writing Group for the PEPI Trial, "Effects of estrogen or estrogen/progestin regimens on heart disease risk factors in postmenopausal women: the Postmenopausal Estrogen/Progestin Interventions (PEPI) Trial." *Journal of the American Medical Association*, 18 January 1995;273(3):199–208.

CONVERSION CHARTS

Metric and Imperial Conversions
(These conversions are rounded for convenience)

Ingredient	Cups/Table-spoons/Teaspoons	Ounces	Grams/Milliliters
Butter	1 cup = 16 table-spoons = 2 sticks	8 ounces	230 grams
Cheese, shredded	1 cup	4 ounces	110 grams
Cream cheese	1 tablespoon	0.5 ounce	14.5 grams
Cornstarch	1 tablespoon	0.3 ounce	8 grams
Flour, all-purpose	1 cup/1 tablespoon	4.5 ounces/0.3 ounce	125 grams/8 grams
Flour, whole wheat	1 cup	4 ounces	120 grams
Fruit, dried	1 cup	4 ounces	120 grams
Fruits or veggies, chopped	1 cup	5 to 7 ounces	145 to 200 grams
Fruits or veggies, puréed	1 cup	8.5 ounces	245 grams
Honey, maple syrup, or corn syrup	1 tablespoon	.75 ounce	20 grams
Liquids: cream, milk, water, or juice	1 cup	8 fluid ounces	240 milliliters
Oats	1 cup	5.5 ounces	150 grams
Salt	1 teaspoon	0.2 ounce	6 grams
Spices: cinnamon, cloves, ginger, or nutmeg (ground)	1 teaspoon	0.2 ounce	5 milliliters
Sugar, brown, firmly packed	1 cup	7 ounces	200 grams
Sugar, white	1 cup/1 tablespoon	7 ounces/0.5 ounce	200 grams/12.5 grams
Vanilla extract	1 teaspoon	0.2 ounce	4 grams

Oven Temperatures

Fahrenheit	Celsius	Gas Mark
225°	110°	¼
250°	120°	½
275°	140°	1
300°	150°	2
325°	160°	3
350°	180°	4
375°	190°	5
400°	200°	6
425°	220°	7
450°	230°	8